Foundations of Applied Statistical Methods

Hang Lee

Foundations of Applied Statistical Methods

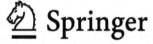 Springer

Hang Lee
Department of Biostatistics
Massachusetts General Hospital
Boston, MA, USA

ISBN 978-3-319-34724-0   ISBN 978-3-319-02402-8 (eBook)
DOI 10.1007/978-3-319-02402-8
Springer Cham Heidelberg New York Dordrecht London

Printed on acid-free paper

Springer is part of Springer Science+Business Media (www.springer.com)

Preface

Researchers who design and conduct experiments or sample surveys, perform statistical inference, and write scientific reports need adequate knowledge of applied statistics. To build adequate and sturdy knowledge of applied statistical methods, firm foundation is essential. I have come across many researchers who had studied statistics in the past but are still far from being ready to apply the learned knowledge to their problem solving, and else who have forgotten what they had learned. This could be partly because the mathematical technicality dealt with the study material was above their mathematics proficiency, or otherwise the studied worked examples often lacked addressing essential fundamentals of the applied methods. This book is written to fill gaps between the traditional textbooks involving ample amount of technically challenging complex mathematical expressions and the worked example-oriented data analysis guide books that often underemphasize fundamentals. The chapters of this book are dedicated to spell out and demonstrate, not to merely explain, necessary foundational ideas so that the motivated readers can learn to fully appreciate the fundamentals of the commonly applied methods and revivify the forgotten knowledge of the methods without having to deal with complex mathematical derivations or attempt to generalize oversimplified worked examples of plug-and-play techniques. Detailed mathematical expressions are exhibited only if they are definitional or intuitively comprehensible. Data-oriented examples are illustrated only to aid the demonstration of fundamental ideas. This book can be used as a self-review guidebook for applied researchers or as an introductory statistical methods course textbook for the students not majoring in statistics.

Boston, MA, USA   Hang Lee

Contents

Chapter 1
Warming Up: Descriptive Statistics and Essential Probability Models

This chapter portrays how to make sense of gathered data before performing the formal statistical inference. The covered topics are types of data, how to visualize data, how to summarize data into few descriptive statistics (i.e., condensed numerical indices), and introduction to some useful probability models.

1.1 Types of Data

Typical types of data arising from clinical studies mostly fall into one of the following categories.

Nominal categorical data contain qualitative information and appear to discrete values that are codified into numbers or characters (e.g., 1=case with a disease diagnosis, 0 = control; M = male, F = female).

Ordinal categorical data are *semi*-quantitative and discrete, and the numeric coding scheme is to order the values such as 1 = mild, 2 = moderate, and 3 = severe. Note that the value of 3 (severe) does not necessarily be three times more severe than 1 (mild).

Count (number of events) data are quantitative and discrete (i.e., 0, 1, 2 ...).

Interval scale data are quantitative and continuous. There is no absolute 0 and the reference value is arbitrary. Particular examples of such data are temperature values in °C and °F.

Ratio scale data are quantitative and continuous, and there is the absolute 0. Particular examples of such data are body weight and height.

In most cases the types of data usually fall into the above classification scheme shown in Table 1.1 in that the types of data can be classified into either quantitative or qualitative, and discrete or continuous. Nonetheless, some definition of the data type may not be clear and among which the similarity and dissimilarity between the ratio scale and interval scale may be such ones that need further clarification.

H. Lee, *Foundations of Applied Statistical Methods*, DOI 10.1007/978-3-319-02402-8_1,
© Springer International Publishing Switzerland 2014

Table 1.1 Classifications of data types

	Qualitative	Quantitative
Discrete	Nominal categorical (e.g., M=male, F=female)	Ordinal categorical (e.g., 1=mild, 2=moderate, 3=severe)
		Count (e.g., number of incidences 0, 1, 2, 3, ...)
Continuous	N/A	Interval scale (e.g., temperature)
		Ratio scale (e.g., weight)

Ratio scale: Two distinct values of the ratio scale are ratio-able. For example, the ratio of two distinct values of a ratio scale x, $x_1/x_2 = 2$ for $x_1 = 200$ and $x_2 = 100$, can be interpreted as "twice as large." Blood cholesterol level, measured as the total volume of cholesterol molecule in a certain unit, is such an example in that if person A's cholesterol level to person B's cholesterol level ratio is 2, then we will be able to say that person A's cholesterol level is doubly higher than that of person B. Other such examples are lung volume, age, and disease duration.

Interval scale: If two distinct values of quantitative data were not ratio-able, then such data are interval scale data. Temperature is a good example in that there are three temperature systems, i.e., Fahrenheit, Celsius, and Kelvin. Kelvin system even has its absolute 0 (there is no negative temperature in Kelvin system). For example, 200 °F is not a temperature that is twice higher than 100 °F. We can only say that 200° is higher by 100° (i.e., the displacement between 200° and 100° is 100° in the Fahrenheit measurement scale).

1.2 Description of Data Pattern

1.2.1 Distribution

A distribution is a complete description of how large the occurring chance (i.e., probability) of a unique datum or certain range of data is. The following two explanations will help you grasp the concept. If you keep on rolling a die, you expect to observe 1, 2, 3, 4, 5, or 6 equally likely, i.e., a probability for each unique outcome value is 1/6. We say "a probability of 1/6 is distributed to the value of 1, 1/6 is distributed to 2, 1/6 to 3, 1/6 to 4, 1/6 to 5, and 1/6 to 6, respectively." Another example is that if you keep on rolling a die many times, and each time you say "a success" if the observed outcome is 5 or 6 and say "a failure" otherwise, then your expected chance to observe a success is 1/3 and that of a failure is 2/3. We say "a probability of 1/3 is distributed to the success and 2/3 is distributed to the failure". In real life, there are many distributions that cannot be verbalized as simply as these two examples, which require descriptions using sophisticated mathematical expressions.

Fig. 1.1 Frequency table
and bar chart for describing
nominal categorical data

Example of Frequency Table

sex	Frequency	Percent	Cumulative Frequency	Cumulative Percent
Female	21	53.85	21	53.85
Male	18	46.15	39	100.00

Example of Bar Chart

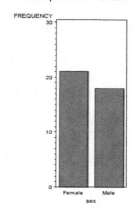

Let's discuss how to describe the distributions arising from various types of data. One way to describe a set of collected data is to make description about the distribution of relative frequency for the observed individual values (e.g., what values are how much common and what values are how much less common). Graphs, simple tables, or a few summary numbers are commonly used.

1.2.2 Description of Categorical Data Distribution

A simple tabulation, *aka* frequency table, is to list the observed count (and proportion in percentage value) for each category. A bar chart (see Figs. 1.1 and 1.2) is a good visual description of where the horizontal axis defines the categories of the outcome and the vertical axis shows the frequency of each observed category. The size of each bar in the Figures is the actual count. It is also common to present the relative frequency (i.e., proportion of each category in percentage value).

1.2.3 Description of Continuous Data Distribution

Figure 1.3 is a listing of white blood cell (WBC) counts of 31 patients diagnosed with a certain illness listed by the patient identification number. Does this listing itself tell us the group characteristics such as the average and the variability among patients?

Fig. 1.2 Frequency table and bar chart for describing ordinal data

Example of Frequency Table

severity	Frequency	Percent	Cumulative Frequency	Cumulative Percent
1:Mild	5	14.29	5	14.29
2:Moderate	16	45.71	21	60.00
3:Severe	14	40.00	35	100.00

Example of Bar Chart

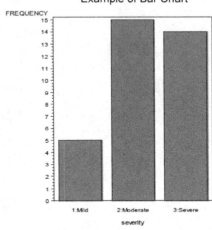

Fig. 1.3 List of WBC raw data of 31 subjects

ID	WBC
1	5200
2	3100
3	3000
4	3700
5	4000
6	3700
7	4100
8	8100
9	3500
10	3300
11	3400
12	9300
13	3800
14	2600
15	4800
16	5800
17	4300
18	6100
19	6100
20	1800
21	7500
22	4100
23	11200
24	2800
25	3900
26	3400
27	8900
28	5900
29	4500
30	3800
31	6500

Fig. 1.4 List of 31 individual
WBC values in ascending
order

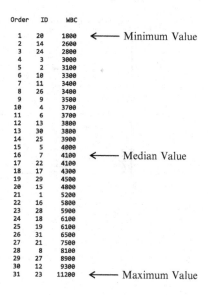

Order	ID	WBC
1	20	1800	← Minimum Value
2	14	2600
3	24	2800
4	3	3000
5	2	3100
6	10	3300
7	11	3400
8	26	3400
9	9	3500
10	4	3700
11	6	3700
12	13	3800
13	30	3800
14	25	3900
15	5	4000
16	7	4100	← Median Value
17	22	4100
18	17	4300
19	29	4500
20	15	4800
21	1	5200
22	16	5800
23	28	5900
24	18	6100
25	19	6100
26	31	6500
27	21	7500
28	8	8100
29	27	8900
30	12	9300
31	23	11200	← Maximum Value

How can we describe the distribution of these data, i.e., how much of the occurring chance is distributed to WBC=5,200, how much to WBC=3,100 ..., and etc.? Such a description may be very cumbersome. As depicted in Fig. 1.4, the listed full data in ascending order can be a primitive way to describe the distribution, but it does not still describe the distribution. An option is to visualize the relative frequencies for grouped intervals of the observed data. Such a presentation is called histogram. To create a histogram, one will first need to create equally spaced WBC categories and count how many observations fall into each category. Then the bar graph can be drawn where each bar size indicates the relative frequency of that particular WBC interval category. This may be a daunting task. Rather than covering the techniques to create the histogram, next section introduces an alternative option.

1.2.4   Stem-and-Leaf

The Stem-and-Leaf plot requires much less work than creating the conventional histogram while providing the same information as what the histogram does. This is a quick and easy option to sketch a continuous data distribution.

Let's use a small data set for illustration, and then revisit our WBC data example for more discussion (Fig. 1.10) after we become familiar to this method. The following nine data points: 12, 32, 22, 28, 26, 45, 32, 21, and 85, are ages (ratio scale) of a small group. Figures 1.5, 1.6, 1.7, 1.8, and 1.9 demonstrate how to create the Stem-and-Leaf plot of these data.

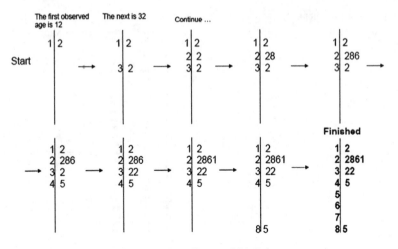

Fig. 1.5 Step-by-step illustration of creating a Stem-and-Leaf plot

Fig. 1.6 Illustration of
creating a Stem-and-Leaf plot

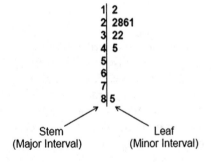

Fig. 1.7 Two Stem-and-Leaf
plots describing the same
data

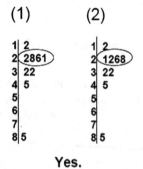

Fig. 1.8 Common mistakes in Stem-and-Leaf

Do (3) and (4) describe the observed distribution correctly?

No. These two showed the stems of 50's 60's and 70's that were described by (1) and (2), i.e., "absence" of such ages.

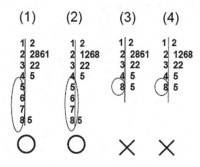

Fig. 1.9 Two Stem-and-Leaf plots describing the same distribution by ascending and descending orders

Are these two describing the same data?

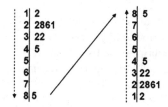

Yes, the plot can be turned up-side-down.

The main idea of this technique is a quick sketch of the distribution of an observed data set without computational burden. Let's just take each datum in the order that it is recorded (i.e., the data are not preprocessed by other techniques such as sorting by ascending/descending order) and plot one value at a time (see Fig. 1.5). Note that the oldest observed age is 85 years which is much greater than the next oldest age 45 years, and the unobserved stem interval values (i.e., 50s, 60s, and 70s) are placed. The determination of the number of equally spaced major intervals (i.e., number of stems) can be subjective and data range-dependent.

As presented in Fig. 1.10, the distribution of our WBC data set is described by the Stem-and-Leaf plot. Noted observations are: most values lie between 3,000 and 4,000 (i.e., mode); the contour of the frequency distribution is skewed to the right and the mean value did not describe the central location well; and the smallest and the largest observations were 1,800 and 11,200, respectively.

```
   Stem-Leaf*                      Frequency**

        11-2                            1
        10-
        9-3                             1
        8-19                            2
        7-5                             1
        6-115                           3
        5-289                           3
        4-011358                        6
        3-01344577889                  11
        2-68                            2
        1-8                             1
```

       *Multiply Stem-Leaf by **1000** Multiply Stem-Leaf by **1000**

       ** Frequency counts annotation is not a part of the Stem-and-Leaf and
       unnecessary but presented to aid the reading.

Fig. 1.10 Presentation of WBC data of 31 subjects using Stem-and-Leaf

1.3 Descriptive Statistics

In addition to the visual description such as Stem-and-Leaf plot, further description
of the distribution by means of a few statistical metrics is useful. Such metrics are
called descriptive statistics which indicate where most of the data values are concentrated and how much the occurring chance distribution is scattered around that
concentrated location.

1.3.1 Statistic

A **statistic** is a function of data, wherein a function usually appears as a mathematical
expression that takes the observed data and reduces to a single summary metric, e.g.,
mean = sum over all data divided by the number of sample size. Note that the word
mathematical expression is interchangeable with formula. As the word formula is usually referred in a plug-and-play setting, this monograph names it mathematical expression, and the least amount of the expression is introduced only when necessary.

1.3.2 Central Tendency Descriptive Statistics
for Quantitative Outcomes

In practice, there are two kinds of descriptive statistics used for quantitative outcomes of which the one kind is the metric indices for characterizing the central
tendency and the second is for the dispersion. The mean (i.e., sum of all observations divided by the sample size), the median (i.e., the midpoint value), and the
mode (i.e., the most frequent value) are the central tendency descriptive statistics.

1.3.3 Dispersion Descriptive Statistics for Quantitative Outcomes

The range (i.e., maximum value–minimum value) and interquartile range (i.e., 75th–25th percentile) are very simple to generate by which the dispersion of a data set is described. Other commonly used dispersion descriptive statistics are variance, standard deviation, and coefficient of variation, and these describe the dispersion of data (particularly when the data are symmetrically scattered around the mean), and the variance and standard deviation are important statistics that play a pivotal role in the formal statistical inferences which will be discussed in Chap. 2.

1.3.4 Variance

The variance of a distribution, denoted by σ^2, can be conceptualized an average squared deviation (explained in detail below) of the data values from their mean. The more dispersed the data are, the more the variance increases. It is common that standard textbooks present the *definitional* and *computational* mathematical expressions. Until the modern computer was not widely available, finding a shortcut for manual calculations and choosing a right tool for a quick and easy calculation had been a major issue of statistical education and practice. Today's data analysis utilizing computer software and knowledge about the shortcut for manual calculations is not important. Nonetheless, understanding the genesis of definitional expression, at least, is important. The following is the demonstration of the definitional expression of the variance.

$$\sigma^2 = \frac{\sum_{i=1}^{n}(x_i - \bar{x})^2}{n-1},$$

where x_i's, for $i=1, 2, ...n$ (i.e., the sample size) are the individual data values, $\bar{x}$ is their mean. The $\sum$ notation on the numerator is to sum over all individual terms, $(x_i - \bar{x})^2$, for $i = 1$ to n (e.g., $n = 31$ for the WBC data). The term $(x_i - \bar{x})^2$ for i is the squared deviation of an individual data value from its mean and is depicted by $\mathbf{d^2}$ in the following visual demonstration.

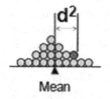

Mean

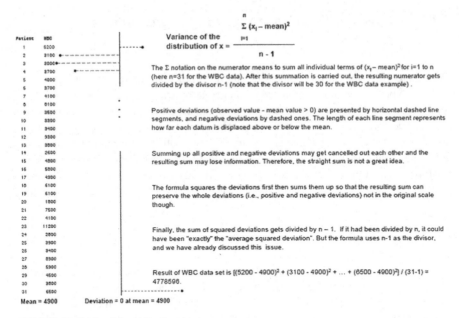

Fig. 1.11 Definitional formula of variance

After this summation is carried out, the resulting numerator is then divided by the divisor $n - 1$ (note that the divisor will be 30 for the WBC data example).

As depicted in Fig. 1.11, positive deviations (i.e., $x_i - \bar{x} > 0$) are presented by horizontal dashed line segments, and negative deviations (i.e., $x_i - \bar{x} < 0$) by dashed ones. The length of each line segment represents how far each datum is displaced above or below the mean. How do we cumulate and preserve the deviations of the entire group? If straight summation is considered, the positive and negative individual deviations may get cancelled out each other and the resulting sum may not retain the information. Thus the straight summation is not a great idea. The individual deviations are squared first then summed up so that the resulting sum can retain the information (i.e., positive and negative deviations) although the retained quantity is not in the original scale. Then, the sum of squared deviations is divided by $n - 1$. If it had been divided by n, it could have been literally the average squared deviation. Instead, the used divisor is $n-1$. Normally an average is obtained by dividing the sum of all values by the sample size n. However, when computing the variance using sample data, we divide by $n-1$, not by n. The idea behind is the following. If the numerator (i.e., sum of squared deviations from the mean) is divided by the sample size, n, then such a calculation will slightly downsize the true standard deviation. The reason is that when the deviation of each individual data point from the mean was obtained, the mean is usually not externally given to us but is generated within the given data set and thus the actually observed deviations could become slightly smaller than what it should be (i.e., referencing to an internally obtained mean value). So, in order to make an appropriate adjustment for the final averaging step, we divide it by $n-1$. You may be curious why it has to be 1 less than the sample size, not 2 less than, or something else. We can at least show that 2 less cannot handle when the sample size is 2, and 3 less cannot handle the sample size of 3. Unlike other choices, $n-1$ (i.e., 1 less than the sample size) can handle any sample size because the smallest sample size that will have a variance is 2 (obviously there is no variance for a single observation)? There is a formal proof that the divisor of $n-1$ is the best for any sample size but it is not necessary to cover it in full detail within this introductory course setting.

The computed variance of the WBC data set is $[(5200 - 4900)^2 + (3100 - 4900)^2 + \ldots + (6500 - 4900)^2]/(31-1) = 4778596$. Note that variance's unit is not the same as the raw data unit (because of the squaring the summed deviations).

1.3.5   Standard Deviation

The standard deviation of a distribution, denoted by σ, is the square root of variance (i.e., $\sqrt{variance}$), and the scale of the standard deviation is the same as that of the raw data. The greater the data are dispersed the standard deviation increases. If the dispersed data form a particular shape (e.g., bell curve), then one standard deviation unit symmetrically around (i.e., above and below) the mean will cover about middle two-thirds of the data range value (see standard normal distribution in Sect. 1.4.3).

$$\sigma = \sqrt{\frac{\sum\limits_{i=1}^{n} d_i^2}{n-1}} = \sqrt{\frac{\sum\limits_{i=1}^{n}(x_i - mean)^2}{n-1}}$$

1.3.6   Property of Standard Deviation After Data Transformations

The observed data often require transformations for analysis purposes. One example is to shift the whole data set to a new reference point by simply adding a positive constant to or subtracting it from the raw data values. Such a simple transformation does not alter the distances between the individual data values thus the standard deviation remains unchanged (Fig. 1.12).

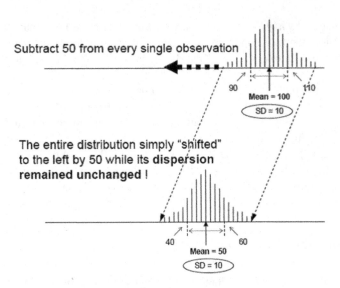

Fig. 1.12 Shifted data without changing dispersion

Another example is to change scale of the data without- or with changing the reference point. In general, if data x (a collection of $x_1, x_2, ..., x_n$) of which the mean = μ and standard deviation = σ_x is transformed to $y = a \cdot x + b$, where a is the scaling constant and b is the reference point, then the mean of y remains the same of $y = a \cdot (mean\ of\ x) + b = a \cdot \mu + b$ and the standard deviation y, $\sigma_y = a \cdot \sigma_x$. Note that adding a constant does not alter the original standard deviation, and only the scaling factor does.

The following example is to demonstrate how the means and standard deviations are changed after transformation. The first column lists a set of body temperature of eight individuals recorded in °C, the second column lists their deviations from the normal body temperature 36.5 °C (i.e., $d = C - 36.5$), and the third column lists their values in °F (i.e., $F = 1.8C + 32$). The mean of the deviations from the normal temperature is 0.33 (i.e., 0.33° higher than the normal temperature on average), which can be reproduced by the simple calculation of the difference between the two mean values 36.83 and 36.5 without having to recalculate the transformed individual data. The standard deviation remains the same because this transformation was just a shifting of the distribution to the reference point 32. The mean of the transformed values to °F scale is 98.29, which can be obtained by the simple calculation of 1.8 times the mean of 36.83 then add 32 without having to recalculate using the transformed individual observations. This transformation involves not only the distribution shifting but also the rescaling where the rescaling was to multiply the original observations by 1.8 prior to shifting the entire distribution to the reference point of 32. The standard deviation of the data transformed to °F scale is 1.12, which can be directly obtained by multiplying 1.8 to the standard deviation of the raw data in °C scale, i.e., $1.12 = 0.62 \times 1.8$ (Fig. 1.13).

Body Temperature °C (Raw Data)	Body Temperature Deviation from 36.5 °C Reference Point (Transformation: $d = C - 36.5$)	Body Temperature °F (Transformation: $F = 1.8C + 32$)
36.40	-0.10	97.52
36.50	0.00	97.70
36.50	0.00	97.70
36.50	0.00	97.70
36.60	0.10	97.88
37.20	0.70	98.96
38.10	1.60	100.58

	Stem and Leaf							

Stem and Leaf	38.(0~4)	1	1.(5~9)	6
	37.(5~9)	2	1.(0~4)	
	37.(0~4)		0.(5~9)	7
	36.(5~9)	5556	0.(0~4)	0001
	36.(0~4)	4	-0.(0~4)	1

100.	6
99.	0*
98.	
97.	0005

* 98.96 was rounded to 99.0

Mean	36.83	0.33 (subtract 36.5 from the original mean)	98.29
Std. Dev.	0.62	0.62 (recalculation is unnecessary)	1.12 (0.62 was multiplied by .8)

Fig. 1.13 Scale invariant and scale variant transformations

Stem-Leaf*		Frequency**
	11-2	1
	10-	
	9-3	1
	8-19	2
	7-5	1
	6-115	3
Mean: 4910	5-289	3
Median: 4100	4-011358	6
Mode: 3500~3999	3-01344577889	11
	2-68	2
	1-8	1

*Multiply Stem-Leaf by **1000** Multiply Stem-Leaf by **1000**

Fig. 1.14 Asymmetrical distribution depicted by a Stem-and-leaf plot

1.3.7   Other Descriptive Statistics for Dispersion

Figure 1.14 illustrates the asymmetrical distribution of the WBC that was illustrated in Fig. 1.10. The mean, median, and mode are not very close to each other.

What would be the best description of the dispersion? The standard deviation = 2,186 which can be interpreted that a little less than thirds of the data are within

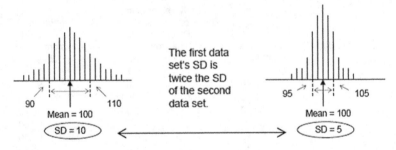

Fig. 1.15 Two data sets with unequal dispersions and equal means

2,714 ~ 7,086 (i.e., within the interval of mean ± standard deviation) if the contour of the distribution had appeared to a bell-like shape. Because the distribution was not symmetrical, the interquartile range may describe the dispersion better than the standard deviation. The 25th and 75th quartiles are 3,400 and 6,100, respectively, and this tells literally that the half of the group is within this range and the width of the range is 2,700 (i.e., Inter-Quartile Range = 6,100 - 3,400 = 2,700).

1.3.8   Dispersions Among Multiple Data Sets

Figure 1.15 presents two data sets of the same measurement variable in two separate groups of individuals. The two group means are the same but the dispersion of the first group is twice as the dispersion of the second group. The difference in the dispersions is not only visible but is also observed in the standard deviations of 10 and 5.

The comparison of the dispersions may become less straightforward in certain situations. What if the two distributions are from either the same characteristics (e.g., body temperatures) from two distinct groups or different characteristics measured in the same unit but of the same individuals (e.g., fat mass and lean mass in the body measured in grams, or systolic blood pressure (SBP) and diastolic blood pressure measured in mmHg). In Fig. 1.16, can we say the SBP values are more dispersed than DBP solely by reading the two standard deviations? Although the standard deviation of SBP distribution is greater than that of DBP, the mean SBP is obviously also greater and the interpretation of the standard deviations needs to take into account the magnitudes of the two means. Coefficient of Variation (CV) is a descriptive statistic that is applicable for such a circumstance by converting the standard deviation to a universally comparable descriptive statistic.

CV is defined as a standard deviation to mean ratio expressed in percent scale (i.e., CV = 100 × standard deviation/mean). This is useful for comparing the dispersions of two or more distributions of the same variable in two or more different data sets of the means are not identical, or those of two or more different variables measured in the same unit in the same data set. As demonstrated in Table 1.2

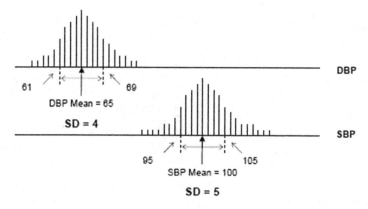

Fig. 1.16 Two data sets with unequal dispersions and unequal means

Table 1.2 Application of CV to compare the dispersions of two different characteristics, measured in the same unit, of the same individuals

	N	Mean	Standard deviation	CV (%)
Body fat mass (g)	160	19,783.28	8,095.68	40.9
Body lean mass (g)	160	57,798.63	8,163.56	14.1

Table 1.3 Application of CV to compare the dispersions of the same characteristics, measured in the same unit, of two distinct groups

		N	Mean	Standard deviation	CV (%)
Body fat mass (g)	Group 1	80	21,118.04	8,025.78	38.0
	Group 2	80	18,448.53	7,993.01	43.3

demonstrates the situation of comparing the dispersions of two different characteristics measured from the same individuals in the same unit. The standard deviation of the Fat Mass in grams is smaller than that of the Lean Mass in grams of the same 150 individuals, but the CV of the Fat Mass is greater describing that the Fat Mass distribution is more dispersed (CV 43.0 % compared to 14.4 %).

Table 1.3 demonstrates the situation of comparing the dispersions of the same characteristic measured from the same individuals. The standard deviations appeared greater within Group 1 but the CV was greater within Group 2 describing that the dispersion of fat Mass was greater within Group 2.

1.3.9 Caution to CV Interpretation

CV is a useful descriptive statistic to compare dispersions of two or more data sets when the means are different across the data sets. However, the CV should be

Fig. 1.17 View of Stem-and-Leaf from above

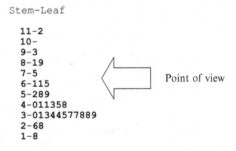

```
Stem-Leaf

11-2
10-
9-3
8-19
7-5
6-115
5-289
4-011358
3-01344577889
2-68
1-8
```

Point of view

Fig. 1.18 Relationship between Stem-and-Leaf and Box-and-Whisker plots

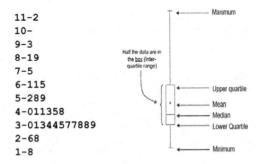

```
11-2
10-
9-3
8-19
7-5
6-115
5-289
4-011358
3-01344577889
2-68
1-8
```

Half the data are in the box (inter-quartile range)

Maximum

Upper quartile

Mean

Median

Lower Quartile

Minimum

applied carefully. When the dispersions of two distributions are compared, we need to ensure that the comparison is appropriate. A comparison of the dispersions of the same or compatible kinds is appropriate (e.g., CVs of body weights obtained from two separate groups, or CVs of SBP and DBP obtained from the same group of persons). However, a comparison of two dispersions of which one of the two is a result of a certain transformation of the original data is not appropriate. For example, in the case of the body temperature example in 1.3.6 the CV of the original °C is $100 \times (0.62/36.82) = 1.68$ % and the CV of the transformed data via °C $-$ 36.5 is $100 \times (0.62/0.33) = 187.88$ %. Did the dispersion increase this large after the whole distribution simple shift? No, the dispersion did not differ and the standard deviations remained the same. However, the CV of °F scale data distribution is different from the original °C scale.

1.3.10 Box and Whisker Plot

Unlike the Stem-and-Leaf plot, this plot does not show the individual data values explicitly. If the Stem-and-Leaf plot is seen from a bird's eye view (Fig. 1.17), then the resulting description can be made as shown in the right hand side panel of Fig. 1.18 which is depicted separately in Fig. 1.19.

Fig. 1.19 Box-and-Whisker plot of a skewed data set

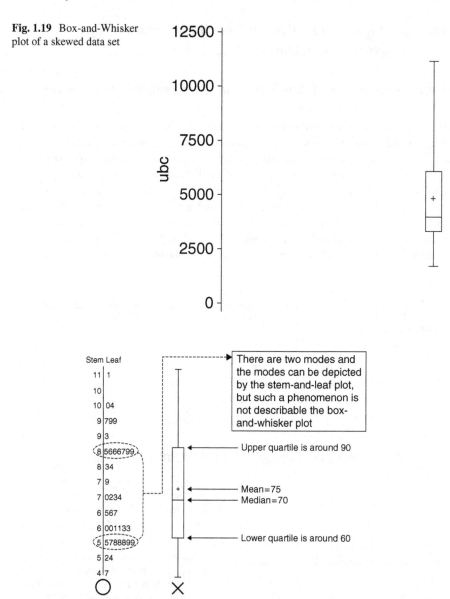

Fig. 1.20 Stem-and-Leaf and Box-and-Whisker plots of a skewed data set

Among the several advantages of this technique, the unique feature is to visualize the interval where the middle half of the data exist (i.e., the interquartile range) by a box, and the interval where the rest of the data by the whiskers (Fig. 1.19).

If there are two or more modes, the Box-and-Whisker plot cannot fully characterize such a phenomenon, but the Stem-and-Leaf does (see Fig. 1.20).

1.4   Descriptive Statistics for Describing Relationships Between Two Outcomes

1.4.1   Linear Correlation Between Two Continuous Outcomes

Previous sections discussed how to summarize the data observed from a single variable (*aka* univariate). This section discusses how to describe a relationship between a set of pairs of continuous outcomes (e.g., a collection of heights measured from biological mother and her daughter pairs). The easiest way to describe such a pattern is to create a scatter plot of the paired data (Fig. 1.21). Correlation coefficient, ρ, is a descriptive statistic that summarizes the direction and strength of a linear association. The correlation coefficient exists between -1 and 1 (geometry of the correlation coefficient is demonstrated by Fig. 1.22). Negative ρ values indicate a reverse linear association between the paired variables and positive ρ values

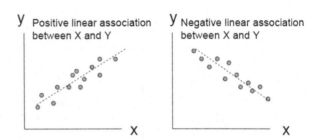

Fig. 1.21 Linear relationships between two continuous outcomes

Geometry and Calculation of Correlation Coefficient

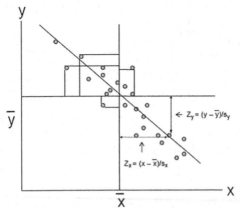

• Measure the standardized horizontal and vertical deviations of individual dots from $(\overline{x}, \overline{y})$, i.e., calculate the z_x and z_y (standardized deviation from the horizontal and vertical means)

• Compute the area of each rectangle and put a sign (Quadrants I and III: + and Quadrants II and IV: -). Note: This is the same as obtaining the product of z_x and z_y

• Sum over all signed rectangles, then the resulting value is the correlation coefficient ρ

• The more same "sign" cumulated rectangles, the stronger linear association towards that sign

Fig. 1.22 Geometry of correlation coefficient

Fig. 1.23 Nonlinear relationship between two continuous outcomes

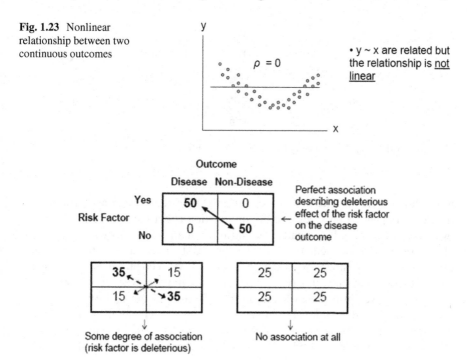

Fig. 1.24 Patterns of association between two binary outcomes

indicate the same directional linear association. For example, ρ between x and y, ρ_{xy} = -0.9 indicates a strong negative linear association between x and y, and ρ_{xy} = 0.2 indicates a weak positive linear association. Note that the correlation coefficient measures only a linear association. Figure 1.23 illustrates a situation that the correlation coefficient is 0 but there is a clear relationship between the paired variables. The computation may be a burden if done manually. Computer software is widely available, and even Excel can be used (see Chap. 7 for details).

1.4.2   Contingency Table to Describe an Association Between Two Categorical Outcomes

Qualitative categorical outcomes cannot be summarized by the mean and standard deviation value of the observed categories even if the categories were numerically coded (i.e., mean value of such a codified data is meaningless). It is also true that an association of a pair of the numerically categorized outcomes cannot be assessed by the correlation coefficient because the calculation of the correlation coefficient involves the mean value and deviations from the means (see Fig. 1.12). A scatter plot is not well applicable for a visual description between a pair of categorical outcomes. In order to describe the pattern of a set of pairs obtained from two categorical outcomes, the contingency table is used (Fig. 1.24, where each cell number

Birth Weight

		≤2500 gms	>2500 gms	Row Total
		Row %	Row %	Row % Row %
Mother's	≤20	10 (20%)	40 (80%)	50 (100% ← 20%+80%)
Age	>20	15 (10%)	135 (90%)	150 (100% ← 10%+90%)
Column Total		25 (12.5%)	175 (87.5%)	200

Fig. 1.25 Exploratory data summary by a contingency table

is the observed frequencies of the study subjects). The number appeared in each cell (i.e., cell frequency) provides you the information about the association between two categorical variables. Figure 1.24 illustrates the perfect, moderate, and complete absence of the association between a disease status and a deleterious risk factor. Figure 1.25 illustrates what data pattern is to be recognized for a summary interpretation. There are 20 % (i.e., 10 out of 50) of mothers who are ≤20 years old delivered low weight babies, whereas only 10 % (i.e., 15 out of 150) of the > 20 years old mothers did so. It is also noted that the 20 % is greater than the marginal proportion of the ≤2,500 g (i.e., 12.5 %) and 10 % is lower than the marginal. This observed pattern is interpreted as a twofold difference in proportion of ≥2,500 g between the two mother groups.

1.4.3   Odds Ratio

Odds ratio (*OR*) is a descriptive statistic that measures the direction and strength of an association between two binary outcomes. It is defined as a ratio of two odds. The odds is the ratio between the probability of observing an event of interest, π, and the probability of not observing that event, $1-\pi$ (i.e., $odds = \pi/(1-\pi)$). In practical application, the odds can be calculated simply by taking the ratio between the number of events of interest and the number of events not of interest (e.g., number of successes divided by number of failures). Thus the odds ratio associated with a presented risk factor versus the absence of the risk factor for the outcome of interest is defined as $[\pi_1/(1-\pi_1)]/[\pi_2/(1-\pi_2)]$. The odds ratio ranges from 0 to infinity of which the value between 0 and 1 is a protective effect of the factor (i.e., the outcome is less likely to happen within the risk group), 1 being neutral, and greater than 1 is a deleterious effect of the risk factor (i.e., the outcome is less likely to happen within the risk group). According to the definition, the odds ratio associated with the mother's age ≤ 20 years versus > 20 years for the offspring's birth weight ≤ 2,500 g is $[0.2/(1-0.2)]/[0.1/(1-0.1)] = 2.25$. The same result is obtained simply by the cross product ratio, i.e., $[(10/40)]/[(15/135)] = (10 \times 135)/(40 \times 15) = 2.25$. The interpretation of this is that the odds to deliver the offspring with ≤ 2,500 g of birth weight among the mothers age ≤ 20 years is 2.25 times of that of the mothers >20 years. It is a common mistake to make the following erroneous interpretation that the risk of having low birth weight delivery is 2.25 times greater. By definition, the risk is the probability whereas the odds ratio is a ratio of two odds.

1.5 Two Useful Probability Distributions

Two important probability distributions are introduced here, which are very instrumental for the inference (see Chap. 2 for inference). A distribution is a complete description of a set of data that species the domain of data occurrences and the corresponding relative frequency over the domain of occurrence. Note that the object being distributed is the relative frequency. A probability model (e.g., Gaussian, binomial model) is the underlying mathematical rule (i.e., mechanism) that generates the data being observed. If you had thought that a distribution is just a curve, or histogram (i.e., visually described data scatter), you would need to revise it.

Two widely applied and very useful models in statistical inference are the Gaussian distribution, a continuous data generation mechanism, and binomial distribution, a count of binary event data generation mechanism (i.e., number of presence or absence of a certain characteristic).

1.5.1 Gaussian Distribution

The Gaussian distribution describes the continuous data generation mechanism, and it has important mathematical properties on which the applications of event probability computations and the inference (see Chap. 2) rely. The name Gaussian is originated by the mathematician Gauss who derived its mathematical properties. Its common name is Normal Distribution because the model describes well the probability distributions of typical normal behaviors of continuous outcomes (*aka* bell curve). This distribution has a unique characteristic that the mean, median, and mode are identical, and the data are largely aggregated around the central location and gradually spread symmetrically. A particular Gaussian distribution is completely characterized by the mean and standard deviation, and its notation is $N(\mu, \sigma^2)$, where μ and σ denote the values of mean and standard deviation (thus σ^2 denotes the variance), respectively.

1.5.2 Density Function of Gaussian Distribution

Density is a concentrated quantity on a particular value of the possible data range of a continuous outcome, and this quantity is proportional to the probability of occurrence within a neighborhood of that particular value. Figure 1.26 describes the

Density Function f(x)
with mean = μ and standard deviation = σ

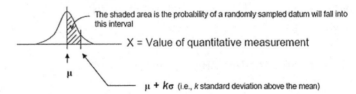

Fig. 1.26 Gaussian density function curve

The proportion to compute is the area under the curve from x = 250 to infinity.

Integrate the density function, which is a daunting task. However **Excel** or other computer programs are widely used for an easy calculation. You will find the answer: top **0.621%**.

Normal Density, f(x), with mean = 175 and SD=30

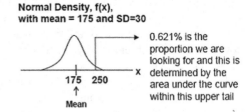

0.621% is the proportion we are looking for and this is determined by the area under the curve within this upper tail

Fig. 1.27 Density curve and tail probability

density of a Gaussian distribution with mean μ and standard deviation σ. The height of the symmetric bell curve is the size of density (not the actual probability) concentrated over the values of the continuous outcome x. The value where the density peaks and the degree of dispersion are completely determined by the mean and standard deviation of the distribution, respectively. The area under the entire density curve becomes 1. As depicted in the figure the shaded area is the probability that the x values exist between the mean and k times the standard deviation above the mean. The area under the density curve from one standard deviation below to above the mean is approximately 68.3 % (exactly 68.2689 %) meaning that a little bit over middle two-thirds of the group is aggregated symmetrically within one standard deviation around the mean of any Gaussian distribution.

1.5.3 Application of Gaussian Distribution

The Gaussian distribution model is very useful tool to approximately calculate a probability of observing certain numerical range of events. The example shown in Fig. 1.27 is to find out the proportion of a large group of pediatric subjects whose serum cholesterol level above 250 mg/mL if the group's cholesterol distribution follows a Gaussian distribution with mean of 175 and standard deviation of 30. Because the standard deviation is 30, the value of 250 is 2.5 times the standard deviation above the mean (i.e., 250 = 175 + 2.5×30). The area under the curve that covers the

cholesterol range > 250 is 0.625 %, which indicates the subjects with cholesterol
level >250 are within top 0.625 % portion. The calculation requires integration of
the Gaussian density function equation. However, we can obtain the result using
Excel or standard probability tables of Gaussian distribution. Next section will discuss how to calculate the probability using the tables by transforming any Gaussian
distribution to the Standard Normal Distribution.

1.5.4   Standard Normal Distribution

The Standard Normal Distribution is the Gaussian distribution of which the mean is
0 and the standard deviation is 1, i.e., $N (0, 1)$. Any Gaussian distribution can be
standardized by the following transformation. In the following equation, x is the
variable that represents a value of the original Gaussian distribution with mean μ
and standard deviation σ, and z represents the value of the following
transformation:

$$z = \frac{x - \mu}{\sigma}$$

This transformation shifts the entire data set uniformly by subtracting μ from all
individual values, and rescale the already shifted data values by dividing them by
the standard deviation, thus the transformed data will have mean 0 and standard
deviation 1.

The Standard Normal Distribution has several useful characteristics on which
data analysis and statistical inference rely (we discuss inference well in Chap. 2).
First, as seen above, the density is symmetrically distributed over the data range
resembling bell-like shape. Moreover, one standard deviation below and above the
mean, i.e., the interval from -1 to 1 on z, covers approximately 68.3 % of the distribution symmetrically. The interval of z from -2 to 2 (i.e., within two standard deviation symmetrically around the mean) covers approximately 95.5 % of the
distribution. The normal range, -1.96 to 1.96 on z which covers 95 % of distribution
around mean, is frequently sought (Fig. 1.28).

Figure 1.29, excerpted from Chap. 10, presents the areas under the standard
normal density curve covering from negative infinity to various values of the standard normal random variable, z. This table can be used to compute the probability
evaluated within a certain interval without using a computer program. For example,
Pr $\{-1.96 < x \leq 1.96\}$ can be computed Pr $\{z \leq 1.96\}$ – Pr $\{z \leq -1.96\} = 0.975 -$
$0.025 = 0.95$.

As shown in Fig. 1.30, the probability to observe a value above 250 if the data
follow a Gaussian probability model with mean of 175 and standard deviation of 30,
then the probability is evaluated by first transforming the value 250 to z value (i.e.,
standardize to mean 0 and standard deviation 1). The transformed z value is 2.5 (i.e.,
$250 - 175 = 70$, then divide 75 by 30 to find 2.5). Finally, the area under the Standard
Normal density curve above 2.5 is the probability of interest. The evaluation of this

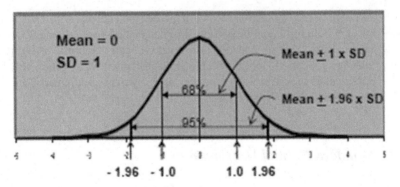

Fig. 1.28 Covered proportions of 1 (and 1.96) unit of standard deviation above and below means in standard normal distribution

Cumulative Probability	Evaluated from negative infinity to			Cumulative Probability	Evaluated from negative infinity to
.	.		.	.	.
0.010	-2.3263		.	0.810	0.8779
0.015	-2.1701		.	0.815	0.8965
0.020	-2.0537		.	0.820	0.9154
0.025	-1.9600		.	0.825	0.9346
0.030	-1.8808		.	0.830	0.9542
.	.		.	.	.
.	.		.	.	.
.	.		.	.	.
0.170	-0.9542		.	0.970	1.8808
0.175	-0.9346		.	0.975	1.9600
0.180	-0.9154		.	0.980	2.0537
0.185	-0.8965		.	0.985	2.1701
0.190	-0.8779		.	0.990	2.3263
0.195	-0.8596		.	0.995	2.5758

Fig. 1.29 List of selected normal random variates and cumulative probabilities up to those values

area can be done by using either of the tables in Fig. 1.29 or any other published tables. To use the first table, we locate the row of the table associated with z value of -2.5 then narrow down to the first column that lists the calculated area above 2.50 (i.e., 0.9938). If z was 2.53, then the fourth column element of the same row would be read (i.e., 0.9943).

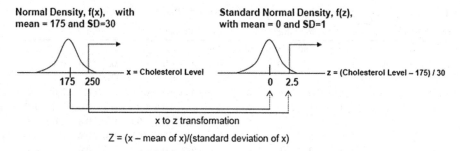

Fig. 1.30 Standardization of an observed value $x = 250$ from N (Mean = 175, SD=30) to $z=2.5$ of the standardized normal distribution, i.e., $N(0, 1)$

1.5.5 Binomial Distribution

The probability values that are distributed to the possible numbers of events counted from a set of finite number of dichotomous outcomes (e.g., success and failure) are typically modeled by Binomial Distribution. For a demonstration purpose, let us discuss the following situation. Suppose that it is known that a new investigative therapy can reduce the volume of a certain type of tumor significantly, and the average success rate is 60 %. What will be the probability of observing 4 or more successful outcomes (i.e., significant tumor volume reduction) from a small experiment treating five animals with such a tumor if the 60 % average success rate is true? First, let us calculate the probabilities of all possible outcomes under this assumption, i.e., no success, 1 success, 2, 3, 4, or all 5 successes if the true average success rate is 60 %. Note that a particular subject's single result should not alter the next subject's result, i.e., the resulting outcomes are independent among experimental animals. In this circumstance, the probabilities distributed to the single dichotomous outcome (shrunken tumor as the success or no response as the failure) of each animal are characterized by Bernoulli distribution with its parameter π which is the probability of success in a single animal treatment (i.e., the two probabilities are π, the success rate and $1-\pi$, the failure rate). The single trial, in this case each trial is a treatment given to each animal, is called Bernoulli trial. The resulting probability distribution of the total number of successes out of those five independent treatment series (i.e., five independent Bernoulli trials) is then described by Binomial Distribution which is characterized by two parameters of which the first is the total number of Bernoulli trials, n, and the second is the Bernoulli distribution's parameter of the success rate, π. In this example, the total number of independent trials, n, is 5 and the parameter of the success rate, p, on each single trial Bernoulli distribution is 0.6. Table 1.4 lists all possible results and their probabilities (0 = failure with its single occurring chance of 0.4, 1=success with its single occurring chance of 0.6). As shown in the last column of the table, these computed probabilities are 0.0102 for 0 successes (i.e., all failures and its probability is $0.4 \times 0.4 \times 0.4 \times 0.4 \times 0.4 = 0.0102$), 0.0768 for 1 success, 0.2304 for 2 successes, 0.3456 for 3 successes,

Table 1.4 *Bi (5, 0.6)*, binomial distribution with n=5 and π=0.6

Number of successes	Result of subjects					Probability
	1st	2nd	3rd	4th	5th	
0 (1 assortment)	0	0	0	0	0	$0.4 \times 0.4 \times 0.4 \times 0.4 \times 0.4 = 0.4^5$
						(Subtotal = 0.0102)
1 (5 assortments)	1	0	0	0	0	$\mathbf{0.6} \times 0.4 \times 0.4 \times 0.4 \times 0.4 = 0.6 \times 0.4^4$
	0	1	0	0	0	$0.4 \times \mathbf{0.6} \times 0.4 \times 0.4 \times 0.4 = 0.6 \times 0.4^4$
	0	0	1	0	0	$0.4 \times 0.4 \times \mathbf{0.6} \times 0.4 \times 0.4 = 0.6 \times 0.4^4$
	0	0	0	1	0	$0.4 \times 0.4 \times 0.4 \times \mathbf{0.6} \times 0.4 = 0.6 \times 0.4^4$
	0	0	0	0	1	$0.4 \times 0.4 \times 0.4 \times 0.4 \times \mathbf{0.6} = 0.6 \times 0.4^4$
						(Subtotal = 0.0768)
2 (10 assortments)	1	1	0	0	0	$\mathbf{0.6} \times \mathbf{0.6} \times 0.4 \times 0.4 \times 0.4 = 0.6^2 \times 0.4^3$
	1	0	1	0	0	$\mathbf{0.6} \times 0.4 \times \mathbf{0.6} \times 0.4 \times 0.4 = 0.6^2 \times 0.4^3$
						(Subtotal = 0.2304)
3 (10 assortments)	1	1	1	0	0	$\mathbf{0.6} \times \mathbf{0.6} \times \mathbf{0.6} \times 0.4 \times 0.4 = 0.6^3 \times 0.4^2$
	1	1	0	1	0	$\mathbf{0.6} \times \mathbf{0.6} \times 0.4 \times \mathbf{0.6} \times 0.4 = 0.6^3 \times 0.4^2$
						(Subtotal = 0.3456)
4 (5 assortments)	1	1	1	1	0	$\mathbf{0.6} \times \mathbf{0.6} \times \mathbf{0.6} \times \mathbf{0.6} \times 0.4 = 0.6^4 \times 0.4$
	1	0	1	1	1	$\mathbf{0.6} \times 0.4 \times \mathbf{0.6} \times \mathbf{0.6} \times \mathbf{0.6} = 0.6^4 \times 0.4$
						(Subtotal = 0.2592)
5 (1 assortment)	1	1	1	1	1	$\mathbf{0.6} \times \mathbf{0.6} \times \mathbf{0.6} \times \mathbf{0.6} \times \mathbf{0.6} = 0.6^5$
						(Subtotal = 0.0778)

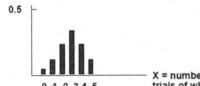

0.5

0 1 2 3 4 5

X = number of success (0, 2, 2, 3, 4, or 5) out of <u>5 independent</u> <u>trials</u> of which the success rate of each single trial is 60%

Fig. 1.31 Distribution (*aka* probability mass function) of *Bi* (n=5, π=0.6)

0.2592 for 4 successes, and 0.0778 for all 5 successes, respectively. General notation of a Binomial Distribution is *Bi (n, π)*, thus in this example it is *Bi (5, 0.6)*. Let us also note that the aforementioned Bernoulli distribution is a special case of Binomial Distribution, and its general notation is *Bi (1, π)*. Figure 1.31 displays *Bi (5, 0.6)*. Thus the probability of observing 4 or more successes out of the treatments given to five independent animals is 0.2592 + 0.0778 = 0.3370. Although this book does not exhibit the closed form equation that completely describes the Binomial Distribution, the following expression can help understand the concept: *Bi (n, π)* can be expressed by *Probability of {no. of events, X = x out of n independent Bernoulli trials}* $= K \pi^x (1-\pi)^{n-x}$, where *K* is an integer value multiplier that reflects the number all possible assortments of the number of success events x ($x = 0, 1, \ldots,$ n). Readers who are familiar with combinatorics can easily figure out $K = n!/[x!(n-x)!]$. In Table 1.4, $K = 1$ for $x = 0$, $K = 5$ for $x = 1$, $K = 10$ for $x = 2$, $\ldots$, and $K = 1$ for

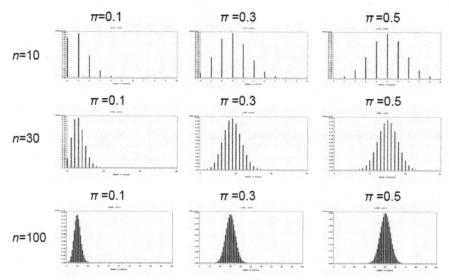

Note: As *n* for a given π becomes large, or π becomes large for a given *n* the Binomial
distribution becomes closer to a normal distribution with mean = $n\pi$ and variance = $n\pi$ (1- π).

Fig. 1.32 Large sample behavior of binomial distributions illustrated by histograms of binomial
distributions with various trial sizes and success rates

$x = 5$. It is straightforward that the expression of *Bi (1, π)* is *Probability of {no. of
events, X = x out of 1 Bernoulli trials}* $= \pi^x(1-\pi)^{1-x}$, where x = either 1 (for success)
or 0 (failure).

   While the Binomial Distribution fits to the probability of success counts arising
from a fixed number of independent trials, if the event of interest is not rare (i.e.,
π is not very small) and the size of the trial, n, becomes large, then the probability
calculation for a range of number of success events can be conveniently approximated by using the Gaussian distribution even if, the number of success is not
continuous. Figure 1.32 demonstrates the rationale for such an application. In
general, for $n \times \pi \geq 5$ (i.e., *the number of expected successes is at least 5)*, if n
becomes large for a given a π, or π becomes large for a given n, then the distributed
probability pattern of Binomial Distribution becomes closer to N ($\mu = n \times \pi$, $\sigma^2 =
n \times \pi \times (1 - \pi)$).

   Suppose that we now increased the number of animal experiment to 100, and we
want to compute the probability of observing 50–75 successes arising from 100
independent trials. Because $n \times \pi = 100 \times 0.6 = 60$, and $n \times \pi \times (1 - \pi) = 100 \times 0.6
\times 0.4 = 24$, this task can be resorted to the normal approximation for which the used
distribution is N ($\mu = 60$, $\sigma^2 = 24$). Then as depicted by Fig. 1.33, the first step is to
transform the interval 50 ~ 75 on N ($\mu = 60$, $\sigma^2 = 24$) to a new interval on N (0, 1),
i.e., $50 \to (50 - \mu)/\sigma = (50-60)/\sqrt{24} = -2.05$ and $75 \to (70 - \mu)/\sigma = (75-60)/\sqrt{24}
= 2.05$. So, the probability to observe 50–75 successes is the area under the density
curve of N (0, 1) covering from -2.05 and 2.05 on z, which is 0.98.

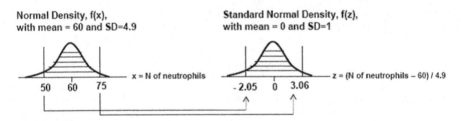

Normal Density, f(x),
with mean = 60 and SD=4.9

Standard Normal Density, f(z),
with mean = 0 and SD=1

Fig. 1.33 Normal approximation to calculate a probability range of number of binary events

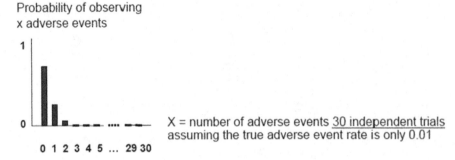

Probability of observing
x adverse events

X = number of adverse events 30 independent trials
assuming the true adverse event rate is only 0.01

Fig. 1.34 Distribution (*aka* probability mass function) of *Bi* (n=30, π =0.01)

On the other hand, when the event of interest is rare and the size of the trial becomes very large then the computation can be approximated by Poisson model in which the number of trials is no longer an important constant (i.e., parameter) that characterizes the Poisson distribution. The notation is *Poi (λ)*, where λ denotes the number of average successes of the rare event out of a large number of independent trials. A particular exemplary outcome that is well characterized by the Poisson model is the number of auto accidents on a particular day in a large metropolitan city. The rare events can be the ones of which the Binomial characteristic constants are $n \times \pi < 5$ *(i.e., expected number of successes)*. The next example is a Binomial Distribution for which the probability calculation can be approximated by a Poisson distribution. Figure 1.34 displays the probabilities of observing 0, 1, 2, ..., 30 adverse events among 30 independent clinical trials of a new drug if the true adverse event rate = 0.01 (i.e., 1 %). The typical pattern of Poisson distribution is that the probability value decreases exponentially after certain number of successes, and as the expected number of successes, $n \times \pi$, becomes smaller the value decreases faster. If we let a computer calculate the probability to observe 3 or more adverse events from 30 trials, then the result will be 0.0033. If we approximate this distribution to Poi (λ =30 × 0.01 = 0.3) and let a computer calculate such an event, the result will be 0.0035, which is not much different from the Binomial model-based calculation.

1.6 Study Questions

1. What are the similarity and dissimilarity between the interval scale and ratio scale?
2. What is the definition of a distribution? What is being distributed?
3. In a Box-and-Whisker plot, what proportion of the population is contained in the "box" interval? Is such a plot useful to describe a bimodal (i.e., two modes) distribution?
4. Please explain the definition of standard deviation.
5. What proportion of the data values are within one standard deviation above and below the mean if the data are normally distributed?
6. Can a correlation coefficient measure the strength of any relationship between two continuous observations?
7. What are the definitions of odds and odds ratio?
8. What are the two parameters that completely determine a Gaussian distribution?
9. What are the two parameters that completely determine a Binomial Distribution?
10. Under what condition can a Gaussian model approximate the proportion of a population lies within a certain range of number of events describable by a Binomial model?

Bibliography

Grimmett G, Stirzaker D (2001) Probability and random processes, 3rd edn. Oxford University Press, Oxford
Johnson NL, Kotz S, Balakrishnan N (1994) Continuous univariate distributions, vol 1, 2nd edn. John Wiley, New York
Ross S (2010) A first course in probability, 8th edn. Pearson Prentice Hall, Upper Saddle River
Snedecor GW, Cochran WG (1991) Statistical methods, 8th edn. Wiley-Blackwell, Oxford
Tukey JW (1977) Exploratory data analysis. Addison-Wesley, New York

Chapter 2
Statistical Inference Focusing on a Single Mean

Statistical inference is to infer whether or not the observed sample data are evidencing the population characteristics of interest. If the whole population data were gathered collectively then there is no room for uncertainty about the population due to a sampling and the statistical inference is unnecessary. It is ideal but unrealistic to collect the whole population data and complete the investigation solely by descriptive data analysis. For this reason, a smaller size of sample data set than that of the whole population is gathered for an investigation. Since the sample data set does not populate the entire population, it is not identical to the population. This chapter will discuss the relationship between the population and sample by addressing (1) the uncertainty and errors in the sample, (2) underpinnings that are necessary for a sound understanding of the applied methods of statistical inference, (3) forms and paradigms of drawing inference, and (4) good study design as a solution to minimize the unavoidable errors contained in the sampling.

2.1 Population and Sample

2.1.1 Sampling and Non-sampling Errors

Let us first discuss several important phenomena and statistical concepts arising from using sample data before addressing the statistical inference. Suppose that our objective is to discover the average (i.e., mean) body weight of a large population ($N > 1$ million) of men and women. It is impractical to measure every individual of the population. Nonetheless, one can probably investigate by using a sufficiently large yet manageable size, n, of well represented random sample. Let's assume that a statistician helped you determine the study sample size, $n = 1000$ individuals of which the sample mean is to serve as a good estimate of the population's mean body weight.

H. Lee, *Foundations of Applied Statistical Methods*, DOI 10.1007/978-3-319-02402-8_2,
© Springer International Publishing Switzerland 2014

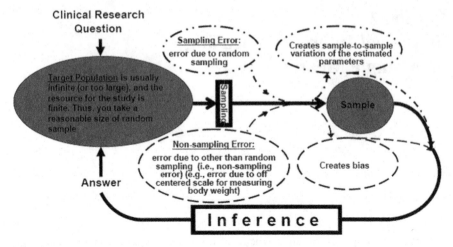

Fig. 2.1 Overview of inference using sample data

The followings are two major sources of uncertainty involved in the sample. The first is sampling error. These 1000 sampled subjects were randomly drawn one at a time and returned to the population (i.e., the chance that each individual was sampled was the same). If another separate random sample of 1000 subjects is taken, then these new 1000 randomly drawn subjects will not be the exactly the same individuals as those initial 1000 subjects. The mean values of those two sets will differ from each other, thus both means will differ from the population mean. A discrepancy between the sample means and the true population mean explained solely by this supposition is understood as the sampling error. This sampling error will eventually disappear as the sample size becomes very large. One extreme example is that if the sample consisted of the entire population, then there is no such an error. The next is non-sampling error. No matter how well the randomly drawn sample subjects represent the whole subjects in the population, it is still possible that there could be another type of discrepancy between the sample mean and true population mean. For instance, if a scale that was used to measure weight systematically underestimated the true value (by accident) because of a mechanical problem, then the discrepancy between the observed sample mean and the true population mean due to such machine error is understood as the non-sampling error. This kind of error will never disappear even if the sample size becomes very large (Fig. 2.1).

2.1.2   Sample- and Sampling Distributions

The concepts of sample distribution and sampling distribution are the important bases of statistical inference. The following example demonstrates the sample and sampling distributions.

The following example demonstrates the sample- and sampling distributions. We are interested in the average neutrophil counts per 100 white blood cells of healthy adults in a large population. Assume that the healthy adults' neutrophil counts per 100 white blood cells are normally distributed with mean of 60 and standard deviation of 5 in this population. Let's also assume that there is no non-sampling error in this sampling.

A random sample of 30 individuals was taken, and the sample mean was calculated. Would this sample mean be exactly 60? Furthermore, if other 19 research groups also had taken their random samples with the same sample size (i.e., n=30) independently, then those sample means of yours and your colleagues will differ. Figure 2.2A.1 illustrates how the histograms of these 20 individual sample sets would appear and Fig. 2.2A.2 illustrates how the 20 respective sample means would vary. A result from the same kind of experiment except for choosing a larger sample size (n=300) is also demonstrated (Fig. 2.2B.1, B.2).

In Fig. 2.2A.1, the 20 sample distributions are described by histograms demonstrating the observed distribution of each random sample set with a sample size of 30 (so-called sample distribution). Each of the other 20 histograms in Fig. 2.2B.1 summarizes each random sample's observed distribution with increased sample size of 300. It is observed that the sample distributions with the tenfold larger increased sample size are more reflective of the population's distribution.

Figure 2.2A.2 depicts the sampling distribution of the 20 sample means in Fig. 2.2A.1, B.2 those of 20 sample means in Fig. 2.2B.1. Note that the observed sampling distribution of the sample means drawn from the 20 repeated samples of size 300 (Fig. 2.2B.2) is much less dispersed than that from the 20 repeated samples of size 30 (Fig. 2.2A.2). The standard deviations of these two sampling distributions provide very good sense of how the sample means vary over the repeated random samplings.

2.1.3 Standard Error

The standard deviation of a sampling distribution measures the variability of the sample means that vary over the independently repeated random samplings. This particular standard deviation is called standard error of the sample mean, $s\bar{x}$. Note that in real life research, it is unrealistic to draw multiple samples in order to describe the sampling distribution as demonstrated in Sect. 2.1.2. The above example was to facilitate conceptualization of the sample- and sampling distributions. The investigators draw only a single sample, and they are not only uncertain about how far/ close the obtained sample mean is from/to the unknown population mean but also cannot produce such a presentation depicted by Fig. 2.2. There is a mathematical equation that allows the investigators to be able to utilize to estimate the standard error of mean based solely on the observed sample data set, which is to simply divide the sample standard deviation, s_x, by the square root of its sample size, n, i.e., $s_x/\sqrt{n}$. In the above illustrative example, a standard error of the sample mean can be

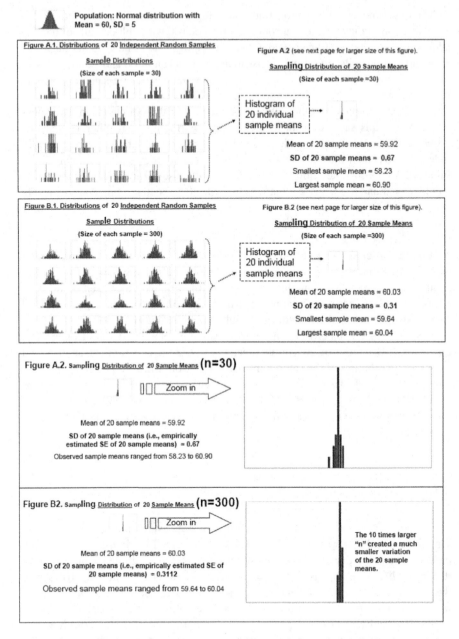

Fig. 2.2 Sample distribution of random-sampled data sets from a normal distribution, and the sampling distributions of their sample means

estimated by directly applying $s_x/\sqrt{30}$ to any of the 20 sample distributions with sample size of 30, which would be very close to 0.67 (or 0.3112 for $n=300$) with a small sample to sample variation. Such an estimated standard error is very close to the standard deviation of the 20 observed sample means from the experiment (such

Table 2.1 Sample- and sampling distributions

	Sample distribution	Sampling distribution
Distribution of	a single sample data set	sample means being obtained over multiple sets of random samples
As the sample size increases the shape of distribution	becomes closer to the population distribution	becomes symmetrical and narrower
Name (and notation) of the dispersion statistic is	Sample standard deviation (s)	Standard error (SE) of mean ($s\,\overline{x}$)
Relationship between s and $s\,\overline{x}$	$s = \sqrt{n} \times s\,\overline{x}$	$s\,\overline{x} = s/\sqrt{n}$

an experiment is called a Monte Carlo Simulation). Table 2.1 summarizes the distinction between the sample- and sampling distributions as well as the relationship between the sample standard deviation and standard error.

2.2 Statistical Inference

2.2.1 Data Reduction and Related Nomenclature

The procedure of the statistical inference can be viewed as an itinerant avenue that connects the sample to population. With a given sample data set, the very first step to walk through that avenue is to reduce the sample data set into several descriptive summary statistics (i.e., extract the summary statistics out of the data set). Such an intervening step of operation is called data reduction. A descriptive data analysis being applied in the sample data for the purpose of making a statistical inference is a good example of the data reduction.

The followings are important statistical vocabularies. A **parameter** is a measured characteristic of a population (e.g., mean age, mean blood pressure, proportion of women). A **statistic** is a measured characteristic as a function of sample data (e.g., sample mean age, sample mean of blood pressure, sample proportion of women). **Estimation** is the procedure to know the value of population parameter of interest using the sample data. An **estimator** is a mathematical function of sample data that is used to estimate a parameter (e.g., $\overline{x} = [x_1 + x_2 + \ldots + x_n]/n$, where $[x_1 + x_2 + \ldots + x_n]$ are sum of all observed values of variable x and n is the sample size). Note that an estimator is also a statistic. An **estimate** is a particular observed value of the estimator (e.g., mean year age estimate = 23, etc., i.e., a resulting value from the data reduction process).

2.2.2 Central Limit Theorem

Central Limit Theorem (CLT) is one of the important theoretical bases for the inference. It describes the typical phenomenon of sample means (the most commonly used central tendency statistic) arising from random sampling.

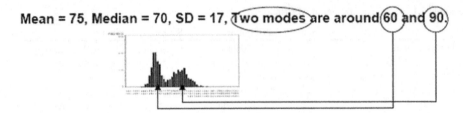

Fig. 2.3 Histogram of a bimodal distribution

The demonstrated sampling experiments below will help the readers understand the meaning and usefulness of the CLT. The next two experiments are slightly different from the ones illustrated in Sect. 2.1.2 in that the population distribution of these sampling experiments is a continuous non-Gaussian distribution. The population distribution from which the samples are drawn is bimodal (i.e., two modes) distribution which often characterizes a distribution as a mixture of two subgroup distributions resulting in two subgroups clustered around two different central locations (Fig. 2.3).

Experiment 1: Draw 30 distinct random sample sets from the given population set with sample size = 25 and make 30 separate histograms for these individual sample distributions. Then make a histogram of the 30 sample means that are obtained from individual sample distributions.

Experiment 2: Repeat the same kind of experiment by increasing the sample size to 100 and create the histograms the same way as the previous experiment.

In Fig. 2.4, as expected, each sample distribution appeared similar to the population distribution, and those from the sample size of 100 resembled the original population distribution more closely. Notably, the sampling distribution of the sample means drawn from the sample size of 100 appeared unimodal (i.e., one mode) and symmetrical (i.e., bell-like) although the population distribution was bi-modal. The dispersion of the sampling distribution of n=100 decreased (standard error decreased from 3.3 to 1.9) which is the same phenomenon that was already observed in the previous experiment in Sect. 2.1.2 (i.e., decreased sampling error for the increased sample size).

Central Limit Theorem (CLT)

For a random variable that follows any* continuous distribution in a population with its mean = μ and standard deviation = σ, if random samples are repeatedly taken over many (m) times independently where each sample size n_k (k =1, 2, ..., m) = n, then the sampling distribution of the m sample means $\bar{x}_k$ (k=1, 2, ..., m) will approach to a normal distribution with its population mean= μ, the population mean, and standard deviation = $\sigma/\sqrt{n}$ as each sample size n increases infinitely.

The sampling distribution of the means arising from a population distribution which does not have a finite standard deviation. One example for such an exception

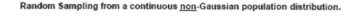

Random Sampling from a continuous <u>non</u>-Gaussian population distribution.

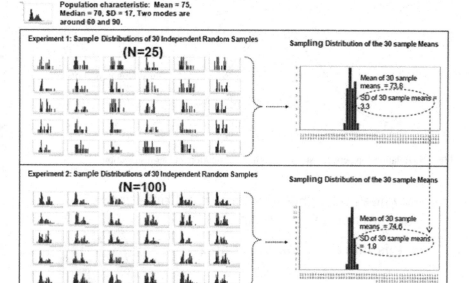

1) With the larger sample size of N=100 the sample distributions became more reflective of the population distribution that is bimodal; 2) The two sampling distributions of the sample means are "bell" shaped.

Fig. 2.4 Sample distribution of random-sampled data sets from a non-normal distribution, and the sampling distributions of their sample means

is the sampling distribution of the means arising from Cauchy Distribution of which the tails of the density curve become much greater, thus the sample means will diverge even if the sample size increases.

2.2.3   The t-Distribution

When the sample size, n, is not large and the population standard deviation is unknown (in many real life studies, the sample sizes are not large and the population standard deviations of the clinical outcomes are usually unknown) the sampling distribution of sample means $\bar{x}$ arising from random sampling from a normally distributed population may not be well approximated by the normal distribution (more spread out than the normal distribution, and the CLT may not be fully applicable), but $\sqrt{n}(\bar{x} - \mu)/s$, a simplified form of $(\bar{x} - \mu)/(s/\sqrt{n})$, where s is the sample standard deviation, is very well described by a t-distribution with $df = n - 1$ (Fig. 2.5).

The t-distributions become very close to the standard normal distribution when the sample sizes are very large (see Fig. 2.6).

Density

T-distribution with *df*=5
(small *df*)

Standard Normal

0.0

-3.0 -2.5 -2.0 -1.5 -1.0 -0.5 0.0 0.5 1.0 1.5 2.0 2.5 3.0

Fig. 2.5 Relationship between standard normal distribution and a *t*-distribution

How does t-distribution with df = n-1 differ from standard normal distribution?

→ t is more spread out than z

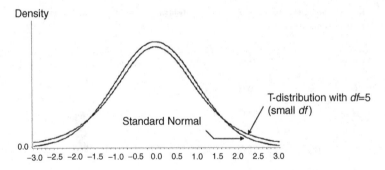

97.5ᵗʰ percentiles of

t-distribution	Standard Normal Distribution
2.228 when df = 10	1.96
2.086 when df = 20	1.96
2.042 when df = 30	1.96
1.980 when df = 120	1.96
1.970 when df = 240	1.96
1.960 when df → ∞	1.96

Note: t-value approaches to 1.96 (i.e., 97.5ᵗʰ percentile of z)
when df = n-1 becomes very large (i.e., ∞)

Fig. 2.6 *t*-Distributions of small and large degrees of freedom versus standard normal distribution

Comment on degrees of freedom (*df*) and beyond: In-depth understanding of degrees of freedom requires ample knowledge of mathematical statistics and linear algebra, and the following is a simple explanation for the applied users. The degrees of freedom, *df*, whenever appears, is understood as a parameter that characterizes a particular probability distribution (e.g., *t*, *F*, *or* $\chi 2$—*will be discussed later*). In practice, finding out the value of *df* is necessary for the inference. The upcoming chapters and sections will focus only onto the minimally necessary knowledge about it while leaving out the details from this book for the statistical analysis package programs calculate the *df*. Besides the degrees of freedom, there is an additional parameter to characterize a *t*-distribution but was not dealt with yet and will be introduced in Chap. 8 because the involvement of non-centrality parameter is unnecessary until the power and sample size topic appears in Chap. 8. Until then, all t-distributions being dealt with are assumed to have their non-centrality parameter of 0 (aka, central t-distribution).

2.2.4 Testing Hypotheses

2.2.4.1 Statistical Hypotheses and Logical Framework of Testing Hypotheses

The main objective of a scientific investigation is to convince that a new discovery is different (improved) from what has been discovered in the past. Scientific investigations usually involve formal procedures consisting of articulating a research hypothesis about the anticipated new finding, design of a study, conducting the study (i.e., experiment or observation) and gather data, and performing data analysis (i.e., make statistical inference) to reveal the data evidence that is beyond the reasonable doubt. The primary reason for performing data analysis is to carry out inference. There are two forms to carry out the inference and they are the hypothesis test and estimation (especially, interval estimation). We will discuss the hypothesis first and then discus the estimation (focusing on the interval estimation).

The hypothesis test requires stated hypotheses (facts) and a test rule, and it can be viewed as a two-player game like framework based on a certain test rule in that the researcher states a pair of mutually contradictory hypotheses of which the first is to be ruled out if data evidence is not strong and the second is to be favorably admitted if data evidence is strong. For example, "a new intervention A is as efficacious as the currently available intervention B" can be such a form of the first hypothesis of the pair and "a new intervention A is more efficacious than the currently available intervention B" can be the second of the pair. Traditionally, the first hypothesis is denoted by H_0 and the second by H_1.

Having stated H_0 and H_1, the next step is to test if the data evidence favors H_0 or H_1 based on a rigorous and objective statistical rule. The test result can either rule out H_0 so that the study can finally pronounce that H_1 wins H_0, or *vice versa*. The logical framework of claiming H_1 given the data evidence is not to let the data evidence prove the proposition H_1 directly, but it is rather to rule out H_0 if the observed data showed a significant counter evidence against H_0. On the other hand, if the counter evidence against H_0 was not significantly strong then this logical framework lets the researcher return to H_0 (i.e., "the past scientific finding remains valid, so go back to the drawing board"). By this procedure a researcher can set H_1 as a new milestone if the data evidence was significant to rule out H_0 (i.e., "record is now broken"). Thus H_0 is called null hypothesis (i.e., back to null) and H_1 is called alternative hypothesis.

In this procedure, the test rule-based final decision is to reject the null hypothesis, H_0, or to fail to reject it. Here, "fail to reject" H_0 is not synonymous with "accept" H_1 in that the observed data cannot be absolutely certain and perfect because the observed sample data always involve uncertainty (i.e., sampling and non-sampling errors), and the sample data can never be able to prove either hypothesis. One may argue why we do not carry out an inference involving only H_1 as the solo player and let the study data directly prove it? Justifications can be made by from purely mathematical to very pragmatic manners. One pragmatic justification can be that H_0 versus H_1 approach always directs the researchers to the next study plan because the approach offers two options of either returning to H_0 or proceeding to with H_1. The analogy is the logical framework of the court room trial. A defendant remains innocent (H_0) if there are insufficient factual evidences, otherwise she/he becomes guilty (H_1) if there were sufficient factual evidences.

2.2.4.2 Step by Step Overview of Hypothesis Test Procedure

This is a *formula-less* overview of the hypothesis test procedure. The flow can be broken down into five steps. Note that such a breakdown is quite arbitrary and made for convenience.

Step 1: Stating null (H_0) and alternative (H_1) hypotheses. This step usually takes place at the beginning of the study (i.e., protocol development stage). The study investigator translates the research hypotheses into the statistical hypotheses and writes them in the statistical analysis plan section of the protocol.

Step 2: Establishing the test rule (decision rule to determine the significance of the observed data evidence to reject the null hypothesis). This step also usually takes place at the protocol development stage. The study investigator articulates the decision rule (i.e., method of a test) in the statistical analysis plan section of the protocol.

Step 3: Collecting data (i.e., conduct clinical study according to the written protocol) and data reduction (i.e., perform data analysis to obtain sample statistics).

Step 4: Applying the rule specified in Step 2 to the results of the data reduction and make decision (i.e., perform data analysis).

Step 5: Making interpretation and report writing.

2.2.4.3 Stating Null and Alternative Hypotheses

The following four sets of null and alternative hypotheses are typical formats of the hypotheses that are written for one mean inference (Table 2.2).

2.2.4.4 How to Phrase the Statistical Hypotheses?

A hypothesis is a statement about a deterministic fact of the population (i.e., not a statement of data being sampled), and the standard format of a written statistical hypothesis is that its tense is present and the words statistically significant should not be in the sentence. Table 2.3 exhibits some examples of improper phrases.

Table 2.2 Null and alternative hypotheses

Null hypothesis	Alternative hypothesis	Simple or composite	Directionality of composite hypothesis
$H_0: \mu = \mu_0$	$H_1: \mu = \mu_1$	Simple null	N/A
Mean is equal to μ_0	Mean is equal to μ_1	Simple alternative	
$H_0: \mu = \mu_0$	$H_1: \mu \neq \mu_0$	Simple null	Nondirectional
Mean is equal to μ_0	Mean is not equal μ_0	Composite alternative	(two-sided)
$H_0: \mu = \mu_0$	$H_1: \mu > \mu_0$	Simple null	Directional
Mean is equal to μ_0	Mean is greater than μ_0	Composite alternative	
$H_0: \mu = \mu_0$	$H_1: \mu < \mu_0$	Simple null	Directional
Mean is equal to μ_0	Mean is smaller than μ_0	Composite alternative	

Note: In some tests, the null hypothesis can be directional and composite. For example, $H_0: \mu \leq \mu_0$ vs. H1: $\mu > \mu_0$ is such a case. For certain tests, $H_0: \mu = \mu_0$ vs. $H_1: \mu > \mu_0$ is used interchangeably without loss of generality. Please consult with an intermediate or advanced theory literature for more exceptions

Table 2.3 Examples of improper phrases for statistical hypotheses

Improper phrases	Reason
H_0: The sample mean is not different from 150	Hypotheses are statements about the population, not the about the sample
H_1: The sample mean is different from 150	
H_0: The mean is not statistically significantly different from 150	The sentence must not include the wording "statistically significantly"
H_1: The mean is statistically significantly different from 150	
H_0: The mean will not be different from 150	The sentence should be written in present tense because it is a statement about the fact of the population of interest
H_1: The mean will be different from 150	

2.2.4.5 Significance of the Test

Having *stated* the null and alternative hypotheses, the researcher collects data that would or would not disprove the null hypothesis. While there are many important constituents of the process, introducing all at once may create confusion. The following discussion focuses onto the significance testing.

Nomenclature

A **level of significance** (or significance level in short), α, is chosen by the researcher before the data analysis (i.e., this is not a resulted value from the observed data), and it determines the resilience of the test rule to reject the null hypothesis. This level is the maximally allowed error probability size that the test would reject the null hypothesis erroneously even though it should not be rejected. Such a decision error is called Type-I error. The level of significance is also called test size. A common choice is 5 %.

A **test statistic** is a sample statistic (see Sects. 1.3.1 and 2.2.1 for its definition) to gauge the strength of an evidence opposing to H_0. Its value is calculated from the observed sample data and it varies from sample to sample (i.e., study to study). The phenomenon of this sample to sample variation of the test statistic is measured by the standard error of the test statistic (i.e., standard deviation of the sampling distribution of the test statistic). The strength of this evidence opposing to H_0 is assessed by the relative extremity (i.e., how unlikely that the calculated test statistic value is observed) of the test statistic according to its sampling distribution (see Sect. 2.1.2 for its definition). The typical (with few exceptions) formulation of the test statistic is constructed by *Observed Estimate ~ Null Value ~ Standard Error (SE)* triplet shown below.

$$Test\,Statistic = \frac{Observed\,Estimate - Null\,Value}{SE\,of\,(Observed\,Estimate - Null\,Value)} = \frac{Signal}{Noise}$$

The numerator, *Observed Estimate—Null Value,* is a gauged metric of the departure of the sample estimate from the hypothesized parameter value specified in the null hypothesis. In this expression, for instance, for a test of which H_0: mean $\mu = \mu_0$ versus H_1: mean $\mu \neq \mu_0$, *Observed Estimate* is the sample mean $\bar{x}$ and *Null Value* is the parameter value μ_0 specified in the null hypothesis. The *SE* is the standard error of the numerator, which is the sampling error of the observed difference of *(Observed Estimate—Null Value)*. The test statistic is the ratio of the former and the latter. A test statistic with its value of 0 indicates the observed mean estimate is equal to the null value, 1 indicates the observed mean estimate's departure from the null value is as large as its average random sampling error size (such a value does not indicate a significant departure from H_0), -1 indicates the same degree of departure from the null but to the opposite direction of the value 1 (such a value does not indicate a significant departure from H_0 either), and three indicates the departure is threefold larger than the average sampling error size (such a large value may indicate a significant departure from H_0) (Fig. 2.7).

Note that this formulation unifies most of the common test statistics for a very simple situation to many complex comparisons situation. This formulation can easily be extended to comparing a difference in two means to a specified null value of 0 (see Sect. 3.1).

Usually the **name of a test** comes from the name of the sampling distribution of the test statistic. For example, *t*-test is the test of which the test statistic follows the *t*-distribution with a particular degrees of freedom (it will be explained later that the degrees of freedom of the *t*-distribution is uniquely determined by the sample size, see Sect. 2.2.4.5).

A p-**value** is the probability of observing the test statistic values that are as or more extreme than the currently calculated test statistic value if the null hypothesis H_0 was true. This probability is calculated by evaluating the tail area under the density curve of the sampling distribution of the test statistic (see Sects. 1.5.2–1.5.4 for area under a density curve). If the *p*-value is less than the significance

Fig. 2.7 Illustration of
concept of test statistic

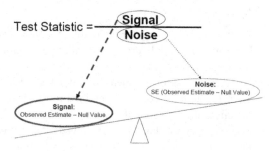

level, α, then it is interpreted that the observed data evidence is significant to suggest that data have not been gathered from the population that is specified by the null hypothesis H_0 (and the probability that such a departure could have been solely due to a chance alone is less than the adopted significance level α). Technically, the evaluation of the tail part area under the density curve will be a daunting numerical integration if a computer is not utilized. However, the idea of resorting to the critical region can replace such a daunting numerical integration. This idea had been applied widely when the modern computer was not popularly utilized.

A **critical region** of a test statistic is a collection of all possible test statistic values (i.e., an interval or multiple intervals of the test statistic values on the sampling distribution) of which the total probability for encountering all such values is less than the significance level when the null hypothesis H_0 is true. The critical region of a particular test is primarily determined by the adopted significance level (i.e., the critical region becomes narrower as the adopted significance level becomes more stringent). H_0 is then rejected at the adopted significance level if the observed test statistic value falls into this region. Note that the critical region is also called rejection region. Checking if the test statistic resides in- or outside of the rejection region can be done using a statistical table of the sampling distribution of the test statistic. The statistical table is a collection of the intervals on the possible range of the test statistic and their corresponding probability of occurrence. Note that if the test statistic value is equal to the critical value, then the p-value is equal to the adopted significance level; if it fell into (outside) the critical region, then p-value is less (greater) than the significance level.

2.2.4.6   One-Sample *t*-Test

This section introduces one-sample *t*-test for the inference about a single mean of a population. The following example is used for introducing the procedure, particularly why this test is called *t*-test, and how the aforementioned constituents covered in Sect. 2.2.4.4 are put into operation in the previously mentioned five steps.

Example 2.1

A laboratory investigator is conducting an animal study to test if a synthetic hormone that is delivered via dermal gel cream applied directly to the thigh muscle of mouse. The investigator hypothesized that the hormone level circulating in mouse blood measured at 1 h after the proper application is about 15 % of the total volume contained in the prescribed gel dose. Furthermore, the circulating hormonal volumes are known to follow a normal distribution. The investigator plans that if the current experiment shows the mean circulating volume is at least 15 % then the gel's hormone concentration will not be increased, otherwise a new experiment with an increased concentration rate will be conducted.

Step 1—Statistical hypotheses are stated
The first step for the hypothesis test inference is to state the null- and alternative hypothesis. The investigational objective can be translated into as below. Null hypothesis: the mean is 15 (i.e., H_0: $\mu = 15$). Alternative hypothesis: the mean is less than 15 (i.e., H_1: $\mu < 15$).

Step 2—Test rule is outlined
A 5 % significance level, i.e., $\alpha = 0.05$, is adopted. The lab scientists would reject the null hypothesis if $p < 0.05$, or equivalently if the observed test statistic falls into the critical region of the test static's sampling distribution (i.e., the test statistic falls outside the interval determined by the 5 % alpha level). The test statistic will gauge the ratio of *(observed mean—null mean) / (standard error of the numerator difference)*.

Step 3—Observe the data
The investigator randomly selected ten mice with the same body weight, and then applied exactly the same dose of the gel to each experimental animal. The following data are the circulating volumes measured in percentage value of the delivered gel volume:
    14.45, 14.40, 14.25, 14.27, 14.57, 14.99, 12.97, 15.29, 15.07, 14.67.

Step 4—Data analysis
The objective of data analysis of the hypothesis test is to calculate the test statistic (i.e., data reduction) and make a decision to reject or not to reject H_0 based on the rule. The rule had been outlined briefly at step 2. With the observed data the rule can be completed now. The first task is to formulate the test statistic and calculate its value. The second task is to evaluate the significance of it either by directly calculating the p-value or determine if it falls into/outside (of) the critical region of the test statistic. The third task is to make decision. The test statistic is constructed as (the observed mean—null value) / SE (of the numerator). The observed mean of the ten observations is 14.493 and its null value is 15. Note that the null value is the

Fig. 2.8 Determination of
p-value of a test statistic in a
one-sample directional *t*-test

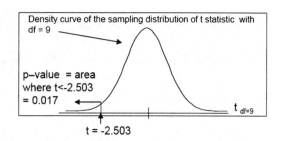

parameter value that is expected if the null hypothesis is true. The numerator part, which is to measure the signal of observed data departure from the null value, is $14.493 - 15 = -0.507$ (approximately half minutes faster than 15 min). The denominator, which is the random sampling noise (i.e., the standard error of the signal), should be sought. Note that the null value is a fixed constant and it does not add additional sampling variation to the signal *Observed Estimate—Null Value.* Therefore, the standard error of the whole numerator remains the same as that of only the observed sample mean. The standard error of the observed sample mean can be calculated by dividing the sample standard deviation by the square root of the sample size (see Sect. 2.1.3). The sample standard deviation is 0.640, thus the standard error is $0.640/\sqrt{10} = 0.203$. Finally the test statistic value is obtained, i.e., $-0.507/0.203 = -2.503$. Let's take a close look of the test statistic. The mathematical expression of this test statistics is congruent to the quantity $(\bar{x} - \mu)/(s/\sqrt{n})$ that follows a *t-distribution* introduced in Sect. 2.2.3, where $\bar{x} - \mu$ is the notational expression of numerator of the test statistic and $(s/\sqrt{n})$ is that of its denominator. The test statistic will follow a *t*-distribution with $df = n-1$, where *n* is the sample size, and if the raw data were from a normally distributed population. Thus the test statistic calculated from these data will follow the *t*-distribution with $df = 10 - 1 = 9$. The naming convention of a test is to give the name of the sampling distribution of the test statistic. Having known the sampling distribution of this test statistic is *t*-distribution, we call this a *t*-test. It is worth mentioning here at least briefly that test statistics can be derived from many situations that are not exactly the same as the above inference (i.e., testing if a single mean is equal to a particular value). For example, a test can be devised in order to compare two means. As we will mention such a situation and other variants in the later chapters (e.g., independent samples *t*-test, paired samples *t*-test), the there are test statistics derived from various situations that will also follow *t*-distribution. In order to uniquely identify the *t*-test being applied to this single mean inference illustrative example, we specifically identify the *t*-test applied to a single mean inference as one-sample *t*-test.

Lastly, we can calculate the *p*-value determined by the test statistic value $t = -2.503$ based on the *t*-distribution with its $df = 9$ (see Fig. 2.8). This calculation can be carried out by using Excel's TDIST function, which delivers a calculated value of an area under *t*-distribution's density curve's upper tail or both tails specified by the user. The user specification, TDIST($|t|$, *df*, 1 or 2), includes the absolute value of the *t*-statistic value, *df*, and the choice of 1- or 2-tail in this order. For this exercise,

	A	B	C
1	One-sample t-test example		
2		Time Length	How to enter / calculate
3		14.45	Enter raw data
4		14.40	Enter raw data
5		14.25	Enter raw data
6		14.27	Enter raw data
7		14.57	Enter raw data
8		14.99	Enter raw data
9		12.97	Enter raw data
10		15.29	Enter raw data
11		15.07	Enter raw data
12		14.67	Enter raw data
13			
14	n=	10	COUNT(B3:B12)
15	Mean=	14.493	AVERAGE(B3:B12)
16	SD=	0.640	STDEV(B3:B12)
17	SE=	0.203	B16/SQRT(B14)
18			
19	H0:	μ = 15	
20	H1:	μ < 15	
21	Mean - 15 =	-0.507	B15 - 15
22	SE(Mean - 15)=	0.203	B17
23			
24	t=	-2.503	B21/B22
25	df=	9	B14-1
26	p=	0.017	TDIST(ABS(B24), B25, 1)
27			

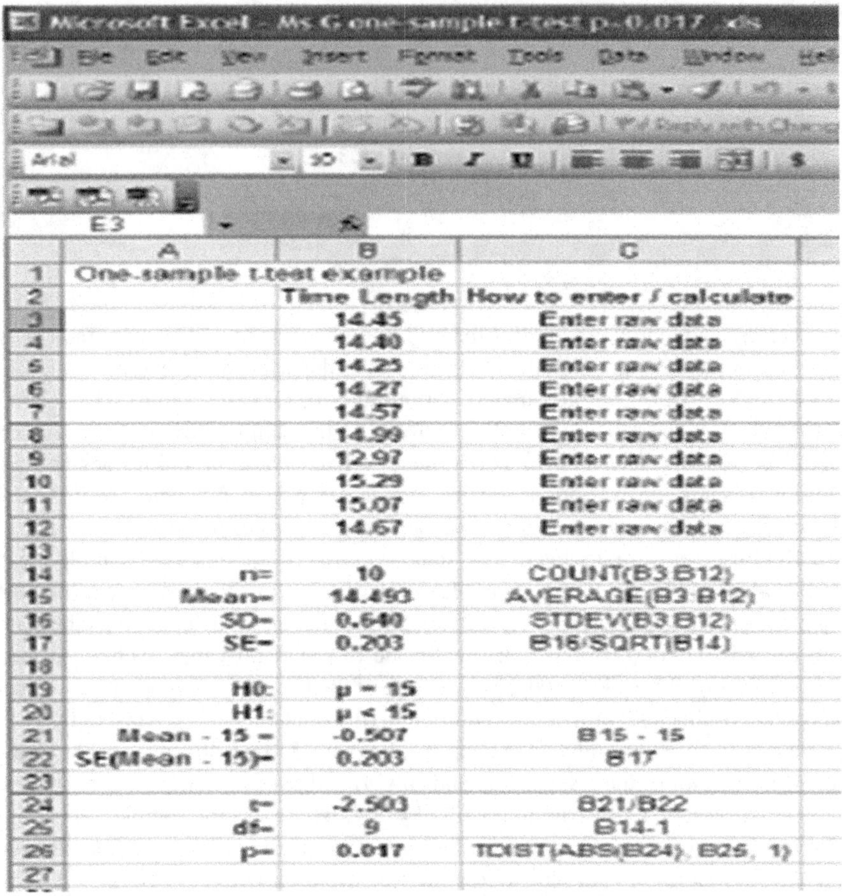

Fig. 2.9 Numerical illustration of calculating test statistic in a one-sample *t*-test

TDIST(| − 2.503|, 9, 1) is necessary. Note that the first input value of | − 2.503| should be either 2.503 (i.e., without notation) or ABS(− 2.503) because the computer program utilizes the symmetrical feature of *t*-distributions. The actual code is TDIST(2.503, 9, 1). Figure 2.9 illustrates how the raw data are organized, the sample mean and its standard error as well as the *t*-statistic are calculated, and how the *p*-value is obtained. The calculated *p*-value =0.017 is much less than the significance level 0.05. Therefore, H_0 is rejected.

We can also take an approach to check if the $t = -3.33$ falls into or outside of the critical region. Figure 2.10 visualize the critical region for this directional one-sample *t*-test on the density curve of the sampling distribution of the test statistic *t* at 5 % significance level. This critical region is where the test statistic is less than the fifth percentile of the *t* (*df*=9) distribution. This fifth percentile is called the critical value and can be found from the *t*-distribution table with *df*=9 and it is −1.833.

Fig. 2.10 Determination of
the critical region of a
one-sample directional *t*-test

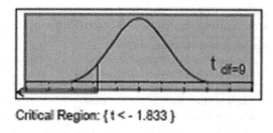

Critical Region: { t < - 1.833 }

The observed $t = -2.503$ is less than -1.833, i.e., it is more extreme than the critical value so fell into the critical region. H_0 is rejected.

Step 5—Interpretation of the result and its summarization
From the above steps this test can be summarized as "These data showed that the volume of the circulating hormone is less than 15 % of the prescribed total volume at a 5 % significance level."

2.2.4.7 Comments on Statistically Significant Test Results

In a clinical study, statistically significant evidence with a tiny size of the signal may not necessarily comprise a clinical significance. Such a result can be observed in a study with a very large sample size (i.e., unnecessarily larger than the adequate sample size). On the other hand, clinically significant evidence can be statistically insignificant due to an inadequately small sample size or very large data variability. Such a result could have been significant if a larger sample size or better error controls (e.g., better study design) had been considered. Chapter 6 is devoted for an in-depth discussion of such a problem.

Reporting format in the results section of clinical research journals is also important. Table 2.4 shows a few examples of recommended and not-recommended formats.

2.2.4.8 Types of Errors in Hypotheses Tests

Hypothesis tests cannot be completely free of decision errors. The first type of such errors is an error that H_0 was rejected although it is true, and the second type is the one that H_0 was not rejected although it was not true. The first kind is called Type-1 error and the second kind is called Type-2 error.

The adopted significance level of a particular test, α, predetermined by the investigator is the maximum allowed probability size of Type-1 error. The maximum allowed probability of Type-2 error size is called β and $1-\beta$ is called power of the test. Figure 2.11 illustrates the probabilities of Type-1 and Type-2 errors of a test of which the null and alternative hypotheses are both simple hypotheses (i.e., a single-valued hypothesis and the test is directional). As depicted, Type-1 error is the area under the density curve of the sampling distribution of the test statistic within the rejection region under the assumption that H_0 is true. Type-2 error is the area under

Table 2.4 Examples of recommended and not-recommended formats of summary sentences to appear in the results sections of clinical research journal articles

Recommended summary sentences	
"These data showed that the mean is significantly different from 15 min ($p = 0.031$)"	Show the actual p-value
"These data showed that the mean is significantly different from 15 min (p<0.05)"	Simply report that the p-value was smaller than the significance level
"These data showed that the mean is not significantly different from 15 min at a 5 % significance level"	A nonsignificant test result at the level of significance = 0.05
"These data showed that the mean is not significantly different from 15 min (NS a at 5 % significance level)"	A nonsignificant test result at the level of significance = 0.05
Not-recommended summary sentences	
"The null hypothesis is rejected because the p<0.05. These data showed that the mean is significantly different from 15 min ($p = 0.031$)"	Do not say in the report " ... the null hypothesis was rejected because p<0.05 ..." Story telling of technical details of the procedure is unnecessary
"These data showed that the mean is not significantly different from 15 min (p>0.05)"	Do not report the meaningless p-values in the concluding sentences when the p-value is greater than your significance level. However, in tables summarizing multiple results together such format is allowed
"These data showed that the mean is not significantly different from 15 min ($p = 0.278$)"	Do not report the meaningless p-values in the concluding sentences when the p-value is greater than your significance level. However, in tables summarizing multiple results together such format is allowed
"The null hypothesis is rejected because the p<0.05. These data showed that the mean is significantly different from 15 min ($p = 0.031$)"	Do not say in the report " ... the null hypothesis was rejected because p<0.05 ..." Story telling of technical details of the procedure is unnecessary

the density curve of the sampling distribution of the test statistic within the non-rejection region under the assumption that H_0 is not true (i.e., H_1 is true). Chapter 6 is devoted to relate the sizes of these two errors and the sample size, and discuss how to determine adequate study sample size to attain small Type-1 and Type-2 errors (Table 2.5).

Note that the following fire alarm system metaphor helps the understanding of Type-1 and Type-2 errors, level of significance, and power (Table 2.6).

2.2.5 Accuracy and Precision

The concepts of accuracy and precision are illustrated in Fig. 2.12. Player 1 performed more accurately and less precisely than Player 2. Player 3 performed more accurately and precisely than the other two players. This illustration can be

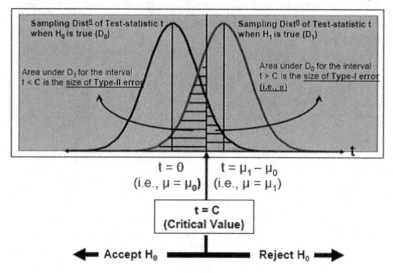

Sizes of Type-I and II Errors
Independent Samples t-test (H_0: Mean $\mu = \mu_0$; H_1: Mean $\mu = \mu_1$)

Fig. 2.11 Determination of sizes of Type-1 and II errors in one-sample *t*-test

Table 2.5 Errors in decisions and their probabilities in a hypothesis test

	H_0 is true	H_1 is true
Accept H_0	Correct decision probability of this correct decision is called operating characteristic	**Type-II error** Probability to commit Type-II error = β
Reject H_0	**Type-I error** Maximum allowed probability to commit Type-I error in a test = α level (e.g., 5 %)	Correct decision Probability of this = $1 - \beta$ = Power

Table 2.6 Alarm system metaphor of testing hypotheses

Hypothesis test	Alarm system metaphor
Type-1 error	Alarm turns on even if there was no fire breakout
Type-2 error	Alarm does not turn on even if there was a fire breakout
Level of significance, α	The level of false alarm system sensitivity
Power, 1- β	Performance level of the alarm system (i.e., turns on whenever it should be) after the sensitivity level is set

considered as three researchers (Researchers 1, 2, and 3 corresponds to Players 1, 2, and 3, respectively) having repeated ten random samplings with a choice of fixed sample size (i.e., n_1 by Player 1, n_2 by Player 2, and n_3 by Player 3) to obtain each point estimate (represented by each "x" mark) using each sample data set and the

Accuracy and Precision

This is a metaphorical illustration (using a 3-player dart game) of the concepts of accuracy and precision of the point estimates.

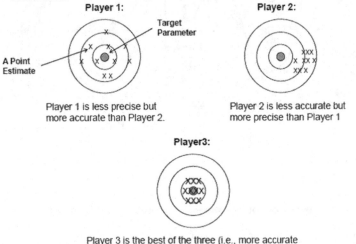

Player 1 is less precise but more accurate than Player 2.

Player 2 is less accurate but more precise than Player 1

Player 3 is the best of the three (i.e., more accurate and precise than both Players 1 and 2).

Fig. 2.12 Illustration of accuracy and precision

same computational method. Intuitively, Researcher 1 might have chosen a smaller sample size than that of Player 2, but might have chosen a better sampling method that prevented the bias that was presented in the estimates of Player 2. How Researchers 1 and 2 could improve their results to expect a result similar to that of Researcher 3? Researcher 1 would increase the sample size without having to reconsider the sampling technique, and Research 2 would examine possible source of systematic non-sampling error and eliminate such cause in the future sampling procedure without having to increase the sample size. Connection of study design and sample size to the accuracy and precision is discussed in Sect. 2.2.8.

2.2.6 Interval Estimation and Confidence Interval

2.2.6.1 Overview

In Sect. 2.2.4 the hypothesis test was applied to a single mean inference. Having rejected H_0 and pronounced that the population mean is significantly different from the null value at the adopted significance level (α), it may be of further interest to find out a set of possible range of the point estimates that would not exclude the unknown population mean so that the interval can be considered as a collection of the possible mean values that are different from the unknown population mean with a certain level of confidence. On the other hand if a test had not been able to reject H_0, could a range be found to include the unknown parameter value? The interval estimation is an avenue to make such an inference, which is linked to the precision.

A popular approach is to construct a confidence interval (CI), which relies on the theory of sampling distribution of the estimator (e.g., sample mean). For instance, the sample mean is a point estimate of the unknown population mean of interest (see Sect. 2.2.1 for the definition of an estimate), and the sample standard error measures the sampling variability of the estimated sample mean. An interval around the point estimate (i.e., the sample mean in the case of mean inference) can be constructed based on the sampling distribution of the sample mean. Section 2.2.6.2 demonstrates a rendering idea of the 95 % confidence interval of the mean while the derivation is illustrated when the sampling distribution is Gaussian with known–unknown standard deviation of the distribution of the population characteristic of interest. The derived lower and upper limits of the interval are indeed the 2.5th and 97.5th percentiles of the sampling distribution of the sample mean and the standard deviation is the standard error of the sample mean. Such a derived interval is one particular case of many intervals obtainable from many repeated random sampling experiments with the same sample size (see Sect. 2.1.2). Of those a large number of experiments about 95 % of the times the individual intervals may contain the unknown population mean. Such an interval is called 95 % confidence interval of the mean.

2.2.6.2 Gaussian Distribution-Based Confidence Interval for a Single Population Mean Inference

If a random of sample of size n ($x_1, x_2, \ldots, x_n$) is taken from a population in which the probability distribution of the population characteristic of interest is a Gaussian distribution with its mean μ and standard deviation σ, then the sampling distribution of the sample mean $\bar{x}$ will follow a normal distribution with mean μ and standard deviation $\sigma/\sqrt{n}$ when n is large (i.e., CLT). Or equivalently, the sampling distribution of ($\bar{x} - \mu$)/$\sigma/\sqrt{n}$ will follow the standard normal distribution (i.e., the Gaussian distribution with mean 0 and standard deviation 1).

One can find out an interval that covers middle 95 % of the observable sample means basing on the standard normal distribution:

Probability $\{2.5th\ percentile \leq (\bar{x} - \mu)/(\sigma/\sqrt{n}) \leq 97.5th\ percentile\} = \{-1.96 \leq (\bar{x} - \mu)/(\sigma/\sqrt{n}) \leq 1.96\} = 0.95$. Then solving $-1.96 \leq (\bar{x} - \mu)/(\sigma/\sqrt{n}) \leq 1.96$ for μ will offer the expression to obtain the 95 % confidence interval of the population mean: $\bar{x} - 1.96 \times \sigma/\sqrt{n} \leq \mu \leq \bar{x} + 1.96 \times \sigma/\sqrt{n}$. If σ is unknown (it's usually unknown in clinical studies), then use s (i.e., sample standard deviation), i.e., $\bar{x} - 1.96 \times s/\sqrt{n} \leq \mu \leq \bar{x} + 1.96 \times s/\sqrt{n}$.

Example 2.2

A small pilot study of healthy women's systolic blood pressure was conducted. The sample mean and standard deviation estimated from a random sample of ten women are 115 and 10.31, respectively. What is the 95 % confidence interval of the mean systolic blood pressure of this healthy women population?

$\bar{x} = 115$, and the population standard deviation is unknown, thus the sample standard deviation will be used for calculating the standard error, i.e., $s/\sqrt{n} = 10.31/\sqrt{10} = 3.26$.

$$95 \% \text{ CI} = (115 - 1.96 \times 3.26, 115 + 1.96 \times 3.26)$$
$$= (115 - 6.39, 115 + 6.39)$$
$$= (108.61, 121.39)$$

Results summary: These data showed that the estimated mean systolic blood pressure was 115 mmHg (95 % CI: 108.61~121.39). Note that the format of this sentence is mostly recommended in applied research articles.

Note that 115 ± 6.39 is not a confidence interval, but is just an arithmetic expression.

It may be skeptical if the sample size of 10 may not be sufficiently large to assume the sampling distribution of the sample mean with unknown population standard deviation (i.e., to resort to the CLT). Alternatively a *t*-distribution can be applied in that the 2.5th and 95th percentiles of the *t*-distribution with $df = n - 1 = 10 - 1 = 9$ are -2.685 and 2.685, respectively (see Sect. 2.2.3 for *df*). Thus the resulting distribution 95 % confidence interval is slightly wider.

Let us discuss how to report the result of interval estimation and why a certain phrasing is recommended. Once a confidence interval (CI) has been constructed, the true parameter (e.g., the mean) is either within or outside this interval (i.e., the parameter is not a moving target but a fixed constant, and the constructed interval is a varying interval depending on the sampled data). The probabilistic argument makes sense only prior to the construction of the CI. If many equal-sized random samplings are conducted independently from a normally distributed population, then the sample means of these random sample sets will form a normal distribution (i.e., the sampling distribution). If we obtain sample mean $-1.96 \times$ SE ~ sample mean $+ 1.96 \times$ SE from each sample (i.e., a 95 % CI based on the normal approximation), then each interval can either include or exclude the true population mean (Fig. 2.13). What's being probabilistic is that about 95 % of these anticipated intervals will include the true mean. And this argument will not make sense once a researcher's sample data already produced a confidence interval. What has already happened is this interval either did or did not include the unknown population value. So, it is not said that "We are 95 % confident ..." but said to focus onto the point estimate accompanied with the numerical interval: "These data showed that the estimated mean SBP was 115 (95 % CI: 108.61~121.39)".

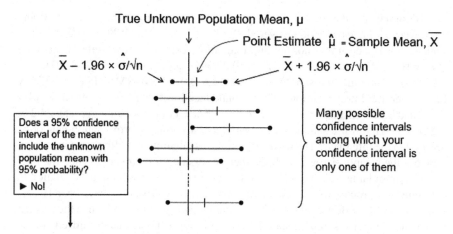

But, 95% of these intervals will include the unknown population mean, and the remaining 5% of them will not.

Fig. 2.13 Illustration of the concept of 95 % confidence interval of a mean

2.2.6.3 Inference About a Single Population Proportion

It is often of interest to make inference about a single population proportion. If we are interested in knowing the proportion of the men and women in a large metropolitan population who were vaccinated with influenza vaccine in the past 6 months, we may possibly take a certain size of random sample of men and women and obtain the information about the vaccination by a survey. The question can be translated into "What is the probability that a man or woman in this population received an influenza vaccination in the past 6 months?" As explored earlier (see Sect. 1.5.5) this question can be well articulated by the Bernoulli distribution in that a single person's survey answer (i.e., coded with 1 if Yes, or 0 if No) being the event outcome and p being the population vaccination rate. We can assume that the answers of the sample of the men and women are independent. The actual inference happens as below. With the sample of n men and women, we first count number of "Yes" answers, which is simply the sum of all 1's and 0's (i.e., $1 + 0 + 1 + 1 + 0 + 1 + 0 + 0 + \ldots$), then figure out what is the sampling distribution of that sum value (let's say it is x). It is obvious that this sampling distribution is $Bi\,(n, \pi)$ and the inference is all about p given n and x.

The inference about p is to find its point estimate, perform a one-sample test if the p is equal to a certain proportion (e.g., H_0: $\pi = 0.3$ versus H_1: $\pi \neq 0.3$), and/or find its 95 % confidence interval. Straightforwardly, the point estimate of π can be obtained by x/n. The one-sample test and the interval estimation can be resorted to the normal approximation (see Sect. 1.2.2) if n is large, or directly to the sampling distribution, i.e., Binomial distribution. For example, if the survey sample size was 1000 and there were 270 persons who answered "Yes" then $\hat{p} = 2705/1000 = 0.27$, the test statistic for a one-sample normal approximation test (i.e., z-test) with H_0: $\pi = 0.3$ versus H_1: $\pi < 0.3$ is $(0.27 - 0.3)/ \sqrt{[0.27 \times (1-0.27) /1000]} = -0.03 / 0.014 = -2.137$ of which the two-sided test's p-value is 0.0163 (NORMSDIST(−2.137) by Excel), and the lower and upper 95 % confidence limits are $0.27 - 1.96 \times 0.014 = 0.242$ and $0.275 + 1.96 \times 0.014 = 0.298$ (i.e., 95 % CI of the vaccination rate: 24.2 % - 29.8 %). What if the sample size is small and a normal approximation cannot be resorted to the inference? The use of Binomial distribution will offer exact inference. Suppose the sample size was only 20 there were six "Yes" answers. Then the one-sample Binomial test H_0: $\pi = 0.3$ versus H_1: $\pi < 0.3$ is reduced into a calculation to determine the probability that the number of "Yes" answers could have been 0, 1, 2, 3, 4, or 5 out of 20 Bernoulli trials if the null hypothesis is true, which is the p-value of the one-sided one-sample Binomial test. This computation can be carried out the same way as what was illustrated in Table 1.4 except for a larger number of assortments of each number of "Yes" answers. Computer program is available for such a calculation. Likewise the 95 % confidence intervals can be determined by finding the 2.5th and 97.5th percentiles of the observed sampling distribution, i.e., *Bi (20, 0.27)*, for which the computation is usually done by computer programs as well.

2.2.7 Bayesian Inference

The aforementioned inference in this chapter, which is called Frequentist's inference, lets the parameter be a fixed constant (not a random variable) and performs either the hypothesis testing (i.e., reject or do not reject the fixed null hypothesis by the chosen rule) or performs the point and interval estimations without the prior probabilistic description about the parameter. Bayesian inference is a method of statistical inference which views the parameter of interest is a random variable (i.e., moving target) and lets the observed data determine the probability that a hypothesis is true. The hypothesis testing in this setting is informal, and the typical format of Bayesian inference is estimation. The word "Bayesian" comes from Bayes, the statistician who popularized the rule (i.e., Bayes' Rule) of conditional probability as described below.

As illustrated in Fig. 2.14, event A can also be conceived as the collection of A overlapping B and A non-overlapping B. The following intuitive algebra is useful for calculating the conditional probability of occurrence event B conditional on A (i.e., event A is already occurred):

$$P\{B|A\} = P\{A \text{ and } B\} / P\{A\} - (1)$$
$$P\{A|B\} = P\{A \text{ and } B\} / P\{B\} - (2)$$
$$\text{From (2), } P\{A|B\} \times P\{B\} = P\{A \text{ and } B\} - (3)$$

$$\text{Plug (3) into (1), then}$$
$$P\{B|A\} = [P\{B\} \times P\{A|B\}] / P\{A\} - (4)$$

Fig. 2.14 Two overlapping
event sets A and B

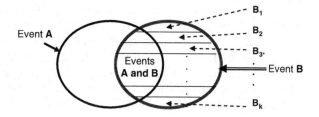

Furthermore, if event B is partitioned into k disjoint sub-events, then P{A} can be reexpressed as P{B$_1$} × P{A|B$_1$} + P{B$_2$} × P{A|B$_2$} + … + P{B$_k$} × P{A|B$_k$}. So, (4) can be expressed as P{B$_i$|A} = [P{B$_i$} × P{A|B$_i$}] / [P{B$_1$} × P{A|B$_1$} + P{B$_2$} × P{A|B$_2$} + … + P{B$_k$} × P{A|B$_k$}], for i (i=1, 2, …, k). Typical application to the Bayesian inference is to consider B$_1$, B$_2$, …, B$_k$ as the hypothesized parameter values and event A as the observed data. Invoking the above facts, we can find out P{B$_i$|A}, i.e., the posterior probability distribution of Bi given observed data, after given the prior distribution (i.e., P{B$_1$}, P{B$_2$}, …, P{B$_k$}) and the conditional probabilities for observing data set A given B$_1$, B$_2$, …, B$_k$ (i.e., P{A|B$_1$}, P{A|B$_2$}, …, P{A|B$_k$}).

Technically, the Bayesian inference picks a prior probability distribution (before observing the data) over hypothesized parameter values that vary with chance (i.e., the parameter is viewed as a random variable) depending on the observed data. We then determine the so-called likelihoods of those hypothesized parameter values using the information contained in the observed data. Finally we determine the likelihoods that are expected over the prior distribution, which is called "posterior" probabilities of the hypotheses. The ultimate decision is to pick the hypothesized parameter value that gained the greatest posterior probability and identify the narrowest interval the covers 95 % of the posterior distribution (i.e., Bayesian 95 % confidence interval).

Following example demonstrates how the Bayesian estimation is different from the Frequentist's estimation.

Example 2.3

A cross-sectional study of estimating the prevalence rate of osteoporosis in an elderly women (age 65+ years) population. The sample size was 500 and the observed number of subjects with osteoporosis diagnosis was 159.

The Frequentist's inference approach to this problem is to find out the point estimate and its 95 % confidence interval based on the normal approximation of the sampling distribution of the estimated proportion. The point estimate is 0.32 (i.e., 159/500). The upper and lower limits of its 95 % CI are $(1596/5000) \pm 1.96 \times \sqrt{[(159/500)(1 - 159/500) / 500]}$, thereby the 95 % CI: 0.28 ~ 0.36.

Bayesian approach to construct a 95 % confidence interval is different as described in a few steps below. Step 1. The investigator views the population prevalence rate is a random variable (i.e., the prevalence rate can vary with chance) that varies within [0.01, 1.00) interval. This is articulated as the "prior" (i.e., prior to data collection) distribution of the population prevalence rate is uniform distribution (i.e., the prior probability for each prevalence rate is equally likely within this interval). Step 2. Invoking Bayes' rule, i.e., the [posterior probability of population prevalence = π] = [prior probability of population prevalence = π] × [probability of observing 159 cases out of 500 random-sampled subjects if π is the true value of population prevalence]. According to the theory the posterior probability is proportional to (not always equal to because the actual likelihood evaluation may take place only within a selective subset of all possible parameter values) the product of these two quantities. Note that there are infinitely many values within [0.01, 1.00) and the researcher may get to evaluate only 99 equally spaced discrete values, e.g., 0.01, 0.02, ..., 0.99, and such a computed probability at each discrete value π is called "likelihood." Step 3. The ultimate goal is to find the prevalence rate that gives the greatest posterior probability and to construct the narrowest interval that covers 95 % of the posterior distribution.

The estimated π of 0.32 is the Bayesian estimate that had greatest posterior probability. In order to construct a Bayesian confidence interval, let's note that the sum of column 5 in Table 2.7 is not 1 but 0.002 because the likelihood value was obtained only within 99 values of all possible values, and that according to the theory the posterior distribution is proportional to the calculated value of the last column. Note that the posterior distribution standardizes the last column so that the sum of those 99 posterior probability values can be a probability distribution (i.e., to make the sum = 1). Because the sum of column 5 is 0.002, we can divide every posterior probability value by 0.002.

The interval that is close to 95 % around the Bayesian point estimate 0.32 (i.e., find where the 95 % of the posterior probabilities are distributed around the point estimate) can now be found out. The values of [posterior probability]/0.002 for hypothesized prevalence value for the following values which cover about 95 % of the posterior distribution are listed in Table 2.8.

The meaning of the Frequentist's confidence interval might not have been very clear (see Sect. 2.2.6.2). However, having appreciated the meaning of the Bayesian confidence interval can be helpful to dissolve such a difficulty. The Bayesian 95 % CI is the interval where the 95 % of the actual posterior probability is distributed, thus this CI is interpreted as "based on the observed data we are 95 % confident that the unknown true and varying population parameter exists in this interval" whereas the Frequentist's confidence interval is not such an interval as we discussed in the earlier part of this chapter.

2.2.8   Study Design and Its Impact to Accuracy and Precision

Good study designs will minimize sampling errors (i.e., increase precision) and non-sampling errors (i.e., increase accuracy and decrease bias) (Fig. 2.15).

Table 2.7 Distribution of posterior probabilities

Hypothesized range of π	Picked value for likelihood evaluation, π^*	Prior probability	Probability of observing 159 cases out of 500 random-sampled subjects if the population prevalence $= \pi^*$ is true	Posterior probability which is proportional to [Prior probability] × [Probability of observing 159 cases out of 500 random sampled subjects if the population prevalence $= \pi^*$ is true]
$0.01 \leq \pi < 0.02$	0.01	$1/99 = 0.010$	$_{500}C_{150}(0.01)^{150}(1-0.01)^{(500-150)} = 0.0000$	$(1/99) \times {}_{500}C_{150}(0.01)^{150}(1-0.01)^{(500-150)} = 0.000$
$0.02 \leq \pi < 0.03$	0.02	$1/99 = 0.010$	$_{500}C_{150}(0.02)^{150}(1-0.02)^{(500-150)} = 0.0000$	$(1/99) \times {}_{500}C_{150}(0.01)^{150}(1-0.01)^{(500-150)} = 0.000$
...	...	...	...	...
$0.29 \leq \pi < 0.30$	0.29	$1/99 = 0.010$	$_{500}C_{150}(0.29)^{150}(1-0.29)^{(500-150)} = 0.0150$	$(1/99) \times {}_{500}C_{150}(0.29)^{150}(1-0.29)^{(500-150)} = 0.00015$
$0.30 \leq \pi < 0.31$	0.30	$1/99 = 0.010$	$_{500}C_{150}(0.30)^{150}(1-0.30)^{(500-150)} = 0.0261$	$(1/99) \times {}_{500}C_{150}(0.30)^{150}(1-0.30)^{(500-150)} = 0.00026$
$0.31 \leq \pi < 0.32$	0.31	$1/99 = 0.010$	$_{500}C_{150}(0.31)^{150}(1-0.31)^{(500-150)} = 0.0355$	$(1/99) \times {}_{500}C_{150}(0.31)^{150}(1-0.31)^{(500-150)} = 0.00036$
$0.32 \leq \pi < 0.33$	0.32	$1/99 = 0.010$	$_{600}C_{168}(0.32)^{168}(1-0.32)^{(600-168)} = 0.0381$	$(1/99) \times {}_{600}C_{168}(0.32)^{168}(1-0.32)^{(600-168)} = 0.00038$
$0.33 \leq \pi < 0.34$	0.33	$1/99 = 0.010$	$_{500}C_{150}(0.33)^{150}(1-0.33)^{(500-150)} = 0.0325$	$(1/99) \times {}_{500}C_{150}(0.33)^{150}(1-0.33)^{(500-150)} = 0.00033$
...	...	...	...	...
$0.99 \leq \pi < 1.00$	0.99	$1/99 = 0.010$	$_{500}C_{150}(0.99)^{150}(1-0.99)^{(500-150)} = 0.0000$	$(1/99) \times {}_{500}C_{150}(0.99)^{150}(1-0.99)^{(500-150)} = 0.00000$

Table 2.8 Rescaled posterior probabilities of the prevalence near the 95 % Bayesian confidence interval

Hypothesized Prevalence value			Rescaled (i.e., divided by 0.002) Posterior Probability	
	0.28		0.033	
	0.29		0.075	
	0.30		0.131	
	0.31		0.178	
Interval I ←	0.32	→ Interval II	0.191	
	0.33		0.163	
	0.34		0.111	
	0.35		0.061	
	0.36		0.027	
Interval I covers			→ 93.6% of the posterior distribution	
Interval II covers			→ 94.2% of the posterior distribution	

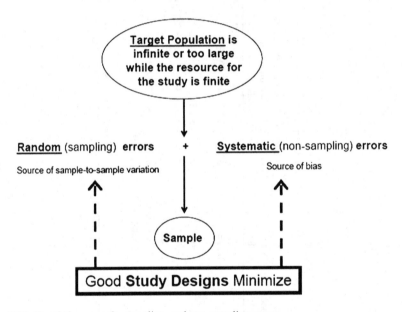

Fig. 2.15 Population, sample, sampling, and non-sampling errors

2.2.8.1   Sampling- and Non-sampling Error Control

Sampling error is the random error involved in the sample statistics (i.e., estimates of the population parameters of interest) arising from the sampling (i.e., sample to sample random fluctuation), and it becomes very small when the sample size becomes very large. An extreme example is that if the observed sample is the whole population, then there is no sampling error (see Sect. 2.1.1). How can a study design control (i.e., reduce) the sampling error? An effort to increase the sample size as much as it can be will reduce the sampling error. Determination of the sample size is a very important part of study design and the ultimate goal is to allow the minimally tolerable sampling error size of the sample estimate to the extent that the investigator can find significant data evidence to answer the study question. However, it is unrealistic to make the sample size very close to that of the population size. Chapter 8 is devoted to discuss the statistical sample size determination based on the statistical power for the hypothesis test.

Non-sampling error is the systematic error that causes the bias involved in the sample statistics due to a poor study design. Unlike the sampling error, it is not sample size-dependent. How can the non-sampling error be controlled? It is necessary to identify the source of it and prevent the bias causing non-sampling error before data collection by making a good study design. There is no simple solution, and developed study design methods are applied for particular situations. The next section will briefly introduce general categories of study types and popular design techniques.

2.2.8.2   Study Types and Related Study Design Techniques

In clinical research setting, studies can be categorized into either observational or experimental study. In the observational study, the outcome causing factors are not controlled by the study investigator. For example, in a study of gender difference in health seeking behavior the researchers cannot assign sex to the study subject because the sex is not a condition that can be created by the researcher. On the other hand, in the experimental studies the study investigator controls the outcome causing factor. For example, the dose levels of a dose response experimental study of a certain medication are determined by the researcher.

2.2.8.3   Observational Study Designs

Case series design is applied in a small scale medical investigation to describe patient information seen over a relatively short period of time. This is a purely descriptive study design, and it does not involve group comparisons and there are no control subjects. Because of such a descriptive nature, this design does not propose hypotheses. The result of a study by this design cannot be generalized.

Cross-sectional design is a technique to examine a selected sample of subjects from a defined population at one point in time. The examples are disease diagnostic test performance study, opinion survey in an election year, etc. Such a design cannot serve as a good design to investigate a causal determinant of the outcome because it takes time for a resulting outcome is manifested by its causal factor.

Table 2.9 Comparison of advantages (+) and disadvantages (−) between cohort and case–control designs

	Cohort design		Case–control design
−	Long study period	+	Short study period
−	Very costly	+	Relatively inexpensive
−	Suitable for relatively common disease	+	Suitable for rare disease
+	Less selection bias in control group	−	Selection bias in control group
+	No recall bias	−	Recall bias in both case and control groups
−	Direct monitoring of study volunteers is needed	+	Medical chart review (only paper documents or computer records) is possible
−	Attrition problem	+	No attrition problems
+	Incidence rates (i.e., probability of an outcome within a certain period of time, e.g., annual cancer incidence rate) can be determined	−	Cannot determine incidence rate
+	Relative risk is accurate	−	Relative risk is approximate

Cohort design is employed to monitor the cohorts of exposed (to a causal factor) and unexposed subjects over a period of time and to examine the effect of the exposure on the long-term outcome by comparing the two cohorts. This is useful for studies for relatively common disease outcomes. However, it requires extremely large cohort sizes to study rare disease outcomes and generally requires a long study period. The potential bias can be prevented relatively easily by this design because the inclusion/exclusion criteria to the cohorts can be defined.

Case–control design is employed to overcome the limitation of the cohort design, particularly the long study period and large cohort sizes problem for the rare outcomes. Unlike the cohort design the case–control design looks back sampled cases and controls retrospectively to verify the risk factor exposure status in the past. The collection of sampled rare cases takes place first through large registry, etc. For example, if a cohort design is considered to study whether or not men with BRCA 1/2 mutation has an increased lifetime risk of breast cancer would require large cohorts of cancer-free men with- and without the mutation and must wait until the study observes enough number of cancer incidence cases in both groups for reliable comparison. However, if the case–control design can reduce the study burden by collecting enough number of male breast cancer patients from already accessible large cancer registry that has been established over many decades and the same number of healthy control men then collect their DNA and perform the comparative analysis. Although the case–control design is less burdensome than the cohort design, the chance for bringing in non-sampling errors is much greater than the cohort design. For example, if the exposure is not measurable by an objective biological material such as DNA, then the collection of the past exposure history may induce recall bias (see Table 2.9). Long-term radiation exposure, smoking history, etc., can be the examples of such exposures.

2.2.8.4 Experimental Study Designs

Experimental designs are often employed in order to rule out potential source of non-sampling errors. In clinical research setting, the clinical trial designs are such kinds. Clinical trials are usually applied to evaluate efficacy of new therapy by comparing the average results of the subject who received the treatment and those of untreated subjects whose demographic characteristics and medical history are similar to those of the treated subjects. The comparison can be made by gathering two groups of randomized subjects who received the treatment and did not receive the treatment (or did receive a placebo treatment), aka randomized study. Randomized study rules out potentially the bias causing non-sampling errors. However, the randomized clinical design can be infeasible in some situations when the placebo use is not acceptable (e.g., urgent medical problems that worsen the subject if remain untreated). The single group cross-over design is to examine whether or not the mean of the before- and after within subject difference is zero.

The key elements of determining the quality of clinical trial designs are randomization, blinding (i.e., let the investigator and/or the study subjects not know that the subjects receive until the end of the study), safety monitoring, and the attrition.

2.3 Study Questions

1. What are the mean and standard deviations of the sampling distribution (i.e., standard error) created from the sample means of three numbers randomly drawn from 1, 2, 3, 4, and 5? Note that there will be ten sample means.
2. What are the two forms in the Frequentist's inference?
3. In CLT, what becomes to form a Gaussian distribution when the sample size becomes large?
4. Under what circumstance a t-distribution is resorted (instead of the standard Gaussian distribution) to the inference of a mean?
5. Explain the idea of "*Observed~Expected~Standard Error*" formulation of the test statistic t of the one-sample t-test for a single mean inference.
6. What is the parameter being tested in a one-sample t-test?
7. What is the quantity of the numerator of the test statistic in a one-sample t-test?
8. What is the quantity of the denominator of the test statistic in a one-sample t-test measure?
9. Why the t-test is named as such?
10. Letting alone the statistical significance, how should these three values be interpreted: $t = 1.5$ ($df = 10$); $t = 2.5$ ($df = 10$); $t = -3.5$ ($df = 10$)?
11. Please distinguish between the 95 % confidence interval around the mean and the 2.5th to 97.5th percentile range of a sample distribution.

12. Please criticize the following awkward sentences:

"These data showed that the outcome was significantly different from 50 (p<0.05)." Is the word "outcome" specific enough?

"These data showed that the mean age was significantly different from 50 years." Does this sentence present a p-value?

"These data showed that the sample mean age was significantly different from 50 years (p<0.05)." Was the inference made about the sample mean? No, the inference is about the population mean.

Bibliography

Beaumont GP (1980) Intermediate mathematical statistics. Chapman & Hall, London

Cochran WG (1963) Sampling Techniques (2nd Edition). Wiley, NY

Gosset WS (1908) The probable error of a mean. Biometrika 6(1):1–25

Hoel PG (1984) Introduction to mathematical statistics, 5th edn. Wiley, New York

Hogg RV, Tanis EA (2010) Probability and statistical inference, 8th edn. Prentice Hall, New Jersey

Johnson NL, Kotz S, Balakrishnan N (1994a) Continuous univariate distributions, vol 1, 2nd edn. Wiley, New York

Johnson NL, Kotz S, Balakrishnan N (1994b) Continuous univariate distributions, vol 2, 2nd edn. Wiley, New York

Lindgren B (1993) Statistical theory, 4th edn. Chapman & Hall, London

Mood AM, Graybill FA, Boes DC (1974) Introduction to the theory of statistics, 3rd edn. McGraw-Hill, New York

Morton RF, Hebel JR, McCarter RJ (1996) A study guide to epidemiology and biostatistics, 4th edn. Aspen Publishers, Rockville

Pagano M, Gauvreau K (1993) Principles of biostatistics. Duxbury Press, Belmont

Snecdecor GW, Cochran WG (1991) Statistical methods, 8th edn. Oxford, Wiley–Blackwell

Williams B (1978) A sampler on sampling. Wiley, New York

Chapter 3
t-Tests for Two Means Comparisons

In Chap. 2, the one-sample *t*-test was introduced to test whether or not a single mean of a population is equal to a certain value. Chapter 3 will introduce the extension of the *t*-test to examine whether or not the difference between the two population means is equal to a certain value. Two situations will be discussed of which the first is when the two means are from independent (i.e., unrelated) populations, and the second is when the two means are from related populations.

3.1 Independent Samples *t*-Test for Comparing Two Independent Means

Example 3.1

Does Medication X prevent the low birth weight delivery?

A prospective two-arm randomized controlled clinical trial (Arm1: Medication X and Arm2: Placebo control) was conducted. Because the study design was a randomized clinical trial, the two study groups are independent.

Shown below is the raw data and summary result of a descriptive analysis. Birth weights (lb) of 15 newborns from mothers with Medication X (denoted by Tx) and 15 from mothers with placebo are listed. Let's assume that the data are normally distributed and the dispersions of the two distributions are not much different (Fig. 3.1).

Tx (n=15): 6.9 7.6 7.3 7.6 6.8 7.2 8.0 5.5 5.8 7.3 8.2 6.9 6.8 5.7 8.6

Placebo (n=15): 6.4 6.7 5.4 8.2 5.3 6.6 5.8 5.7 6.2 7.1 7.0 6.9 5.6 4.2 6.8

How can we tackle this problem? The approach to use an extension of the *t*-test will be introduced first, and then the applied result will be illustrated.

H. Lee, *Foundations of Applied Statistical Methods*, DOI 10.1007/978-3-319-02402-8_3,
© Springer International Publishing Switzerland 2014

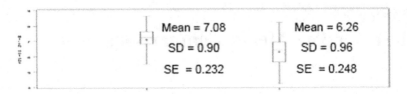

Fig. 3.1 Listed and visualized data from a two-arm randomized clinical trial

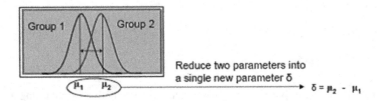

Fig. 3.2 Illustration of two means of normally distributed paired continuous outcomes and difference of the two means

Below is the framework of testing equality of two population means using two independently drawn random samples, both from normally distributed populations. The null hypothesis is that the two population means are equal (i.e., H_0: $\mu_1 = \mu_2$). Note that "two population means are equal" can be translated into "difference of the two population means = 0 (i.e., H_0: $\mu_2 - \mu_1 = 0$)" by which the dimension of the argument is reduced to one (i.e., by letting δ denote the single translated parameter, see Fig. 3.2, where $\delta = \mu_2 - \mu_1$) so that the corresponding sample statistic to work with is the observed difference between the two sample means (i.e., by letting d denote $\bar{x}_2 - \bar{x}_1$). Finally, the null and alternative hypotheses are expressed as H_0: $\delta = 0$ and H_1: $\delta \neq 0$ for a nondirectional test (or H_1: $\delta > 0$ for a directional test examining $\mu_2 > \mu_1$) (Table 3.1).

The idea of "*Observed Estimate ~ Null Value ~ SE* (see Sect. 2.2.4.2)" is applied to derive the test statistic

t = *(Observed Estimate – Null Value)/SE(Observed Estimate – Null Value)*
= $(d - 0)/SE(d)$ (see Sect. 2.2.4.5).

The numerator is the deviation of the observed difference between the two sample means, $d = \bar{x}_2 - \bar{x}_1$, from the null value of the difference between the two population means, $\delta = \mu_2 - \mu_1 = 0$. Note that δ is set to 0 for the equality test. The denominator, $SE(d)$, is the estimated standard error of the numerator. The simplified form of this test statistic is $t = d / SE(d)$. Note that a large value of this ratio (positive, negative, or either direction depending on the alternative hypothesis) indicates that the observed deviation of d from the null value of $\delta = 0$ may not be due to the chance alone. According to the sampling theory, under the null hypothesis and if the two population variances are equal, this test statistic will follow the *t*-distribution with $df = (n_1-1) + (n_2-1)$, where n_1 and n_2 are the sample sizes of the two groups, respectively. We can then find out how extreme (i.e., unlikely to observe) the

Table 3.1 Null and alternative hypotheses for comparing two means

Null hypothesis	Alternative hypothesis	Simple or composite[a]	Directionality of composite hypothesis
$H_0: \mu_2 - \mu_1 = 0$ (i.e., $\mu_1 = \mu_2$) Means are equal	$H_1: \mu_2 - \mu_1 = \delta$ Mean difference is equal to δ	Simple null Simple alternative	N/A
$H_0: \mu_2 - \mu_1 = 0$ (i.e., $\mu_1 = \mu_2$) Means are equal	$H_1: \mu_2 - \mu_1 \neq 0$ Means are not equal	Simple null Composite alternative	Nondirectional (two-sided)
$H_0: \mu_2 - \mu_1 = 0$ (i.e., $\mu_1 = \mu_2$) Means are equal	$H_1: \mu_2 - \mu_1 > 0$ Mean 2 is greater than mean 1	Simple null Composite alternative	Directional
$H_0: \mu_2 - \mu_1 = 0$ (i.e., $\mu_1 = \mu_2$) Means are equal	$H_1: \mu_2 - \mu_1 < 0$ Mean 2 is smaller than mean 1	Simple null Composite alternative	Directional

[a]Simple hypothesis involves a single value of parameter, and composite hypothesis involves more than one value (e.g., an interval) of the parameter

observed test statistic t was, had it been resulted from the sample data gathered from the two population distributions under the null hypothesis.

The derivation of the standard error, $SE(d)$, may seem complex for the beginners. As this book intends not to let the readers plug-and-play formulae, the conceptual steps of its derivations is shown below. The definition of the standard error is the standard deviation of the sampling distribution of a sample statistic (see Sect. 2.1.3 for its definition). The sample statistic of this case is d, which is the difference between the two observed sample means, i.e., $\bar{x}_2 - \bar{x}_1$. So, the $SE(d)$, the standard deviation of the sampling distribution of $\bar{x}_2 - \bar{x}_1$, is to be derived. Because the standard deviation is the square root of the variance, the main derivation is to derive its variance. Note that the sample variances of $\bar{x}_1$ and $\bar{x}_2$ are s^2_1/n_1 and s^2_2/n_2, respectively, where s^2_1 and s^2_2 are notations for the variance of the sample distributions (see Sect. 2.1.2for the definition of the sample distribution). The sample variance of the difference $\bar{x}_2 - \bar{x}_1$ would increase (see illustrative Example 2). Note that $\bar{x}_1$ and $\bar{x}_2$ vary from sample to sample with its variance s^2_1/n_1 and s^2_2/n_2, so the difference $\bar{x}_2 - \bar{x}_1$ would vary greater and the resulting variance of difference is the addition of the individual variances $s^2_1/n_1 + s^2_2/n_2$.

Finally, the denominator of the test statistic is derived, which is the square root of the weighted sum of the two sample variances, i.e., $\sqrt{(s^2_1/n_1 + s^2_2/n_2)}$.

Having derived the test statistic, the inference of Example 3.1 continues as below. The test statistic $t = (6.26 - 7.08) / \sqrt{(0.232^2 + 0.248^2)} = 0.82/0.34 = 2.41$ will follow the t-distribution with $df = 28$. The critical value of this nondirectional test for a 5 % significance level is 1.701 and the critical region is $\{t>1.701\}$. The observed test statistic from the data, $t = 2.41$, fell into the critical region (Fig. 3.3).

The p-value can also be calculated using Excel function TDIST(2.41,28,1), which resulted in 0.0113.

Summary: These data showed that there was a significant effect of medication X to prevent the low birth weight delivery ($p=0.0113$).

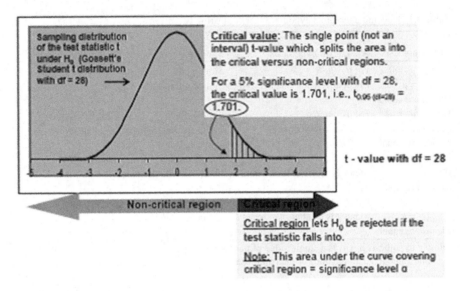

Fig. 3.3 Illustration of the critical region of the directional *t*-test (applied to Example 3.1)

3.1.1   Independent Samples t-Test When Variances Are Unequal

When the two population variances are not equal, the sampling distribution of the aforementioned test statistic will not perfectly follow the *t*-distribution with $df = n_1 + n_2$. This book does not describe computational details but rather devote a conceptual discussion by addressing how we can diagnose such a phenomenon and how we can make inference and interpret the results, provided that the intermediate computational results for the diagnosis and the calculated SE are provided by computer programs or expert statisticians. If the heteroskedasticity was detected, then we resort to a theoretical *t*-distribution with a slightly modified *df*. In this case, a modified *df* will be little bit smaller than $n_1 + n_2 - 2$ than what is obtained under the same variance assumption.

How can we diagnose whether or not the variances are equal before carrying out the independent samples *t*-test? There is a test that evaluates it. The null and alternative hypotheses of this test are $H_0: \sigma^2_1 = \sigma^2_2$ and $H_1: \sigma^2_1 \neq \sigma^2_2$ (note that the nondirectional alternative hypothesis is its obvious choice). Compute the two sample variances and take the ratio of the two. This ratio will follow an *F*-distribution under the null hypothesis. The *F*-distribution has two *dfs* where $df_1 = n_1 - 1$ and $df_2 = n_2 - 1$. Then we resort to this *F*-distribution to determine the *p*-value (detailed explanation for computing a *p*-value from an *F*-distribution will be shown in a later chapter). A *p*-value < 0.05 indicates unequal variances and you would need to take into account this condition during the *t*-test.

Table 3.2 Derivation of the denominator of the test statistic for independent samples *t*-test

Sample size	Population variances	Derived standard error (i.e., denominator of the test statistic t)
Equal	Equal[a]	Substitute n for n_1 and n_2 and s^2 for s^2_1 and s^2_2, so $\sqrt{(s^2_1/n + s^2_2/n)} = \sqrt{(2\,s^2_p/n)}$
Equal	Unequal	Substitute n for n_1 and n_2, so $\sqrt{(s^2_1/n + s^2_2/n)} = \sqrt{[(s^2_1 + s^2_2)(1/n)]}$
Unequal	Equal[a]	Substitute s^2 for s^2_1 and s^2_2, so $\sqrt{(s^2/n + s^2/n)} = \sqrt{[s^2\,(1/n_1 + 1/n_2)]}$
Unequal	Unequal	$\sqrt{(s^2_1/n_1 + s^2_2/n_2)}$

[a]If the population variances of the raw data are equal, it makes more sense to utilize that fact so that we estimate the "pooled" sample variance to derive the denominator of the test statistic. Letting s^2_p denote the pooled sample variance, the weighted average where each weight is one less than the sample size, the result is $s^2_p = [s^2_1/(n_1-1) + s^2_2/(n_2-1)]/(n_1 -1 + n_2-1)]$

If the data showed that the variances are unequal, then a modified version of the independent samples *t*-test is recommended. The main work is to make adjustment of the *df* as well as to estimate the *SE* of the mean difference, which could become biased if not well taken care of. This course material does not introduce the mathematical/computational details. The idea of downward adjustment is that, as the *df* becomes smaller, the tail of the *t*-distribution becomes thicker, meaning that if the *df* is downward adjusted for heteroskedasticity then the observed *t*-statistic will produce a larger *p*-value than that would have resulted from *t*-distribution with the unadjusted *df* because the modified distribution has heavier tail; therefore, the test becomes conservative.

3.1.2 Denominator Formulae of the Test Statistic for Independent Samples t-Test

Other books offer you plug-and-play formulae for calculating the denominator of the test statistic, which prompt you to plug in the sample sizes and the sample variances of the two groups being compared. The readers do not need to drill the computational details as long as they understand the rationale for the above standard error derivation. However, the details are provided in Table 3.2.

3.1.3 Connection to the Confidence Interval

Having concluded a testing hypothesis to merely claim whether or not the two independent means are equal, the researchers may further be interested in estimating the size of the mean difference and its confidence interval. The following numerical illustration is to construct a 95 % confidence interval for the mean difference using Example 3.1 data.

The observed mean difference (i.e., the point estimate of the mean difference between the groups with treatment and placebo) = 7.08 - 6.26 = 0.82 and the

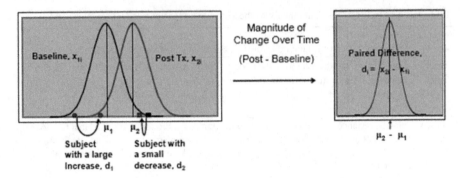

Fig. 3.4 Illustration of distributions of paired normally distributed continuous outcomes and their paired differences

standard error of that observed mean difference = 0.339. The 2.5th and 97.5th percentiles of t with $df = 28$ can be found by using Excel, i.e., TINV(0.05, 28) = 2.048 (or using a table for the percentiles if t-distribution). The lower limit of the 95 % CI based on t-distribution with $df = 28$ is 0.82 - 2.048 × 0.339 = 0.126, and its upper limit is 0.82 + 2.048 × 0.339 = 1.514, thus 95 % confidence interval is 0.126 ~ 1.514. Note that although the test was directional, it is a tradition to construct the 95 % nondirectionally disregarding the directionality of the testing hypotheses. Summary: These data showed that the mean of the treated group was greater by 0.82 (95 % CI: 0.126 − 1.514).

3.2   Paired Sample *t*-Test for Comparing Paired Means

Pairing helps a study design control the subject-to-subject outcomes variation in that the responses to a study medication being studied may vary among different subjects, and testing whether or not the average of the within-subject longitudinal changes in response would eliminate the source of between-subject variation. The following example illustrates the paired sample t-test that is applied to such a clinical investigation (Fig. 3.4).

Example 3.2

Does the use of oral contraceptives (OC) affect systolic blood pressure (SBP)? A self-control (pre- and post-paired measurements) design is applied, and the following test for H_0: $\mu_2 - \mu_1 = 0$ and H_1: $\mu_2 - \mu_1 \neq 0$ is considered.

Following data are the systolic blood pressure measurements in mmHg from ten study volunteers before using OC (i.e., baseline) and those taken from the same ten women after the use of OC for a certain period (i.e., follow-up). Let's assume that the distribution of the SBP values in the population is the Gaussian distribution.

Table 3.3 Sample statistics of the SBP at baseline and follow-up

	Baseline SBP	Follow-up SBP
n	10	10
Mean	115.00	120.40
Median	115.00	119.50
Standard deviation	10.31	13.22
Standard error of the mean	3.26	4.18

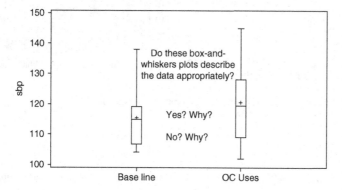

Fig. 3.5 Illustration of inappropriate box-and-whisker plot for paired continuous outcomes data visual display

Subject	Baseline SBP	Follow-up
1	115	128
2	112	115
3	107	106
4	119	128
5	115	122
6	138	145
7	126	132
8	105	109
9	104	102
10	115	117

The following preliminary data analysis (i.e., data reduction) was performed and summarized in Table 3.3. Do these summary statistics describe the phenomenon clearly?

While the summary statistics in Table 3.3 and the graphical display of the data depicted by Fig. 3.5 described that the mean SBP at follow-up was slightly elevated and the variability was also slightly increased, the paired nature of the design was not reflected. Whereas Fig. 3.6 illustrates a typical graphical description of the paired data in that most subjects showed increase in the follow-up SBP and the second panel described that the blood pressure range of the subjects was larger than the average within-subject change.

A significance level of 5 % is adopted. The test is derived based on the "*Observed ~ Null Value ~ SE*" triplet. In order to complete this task, let's revisit the articulated

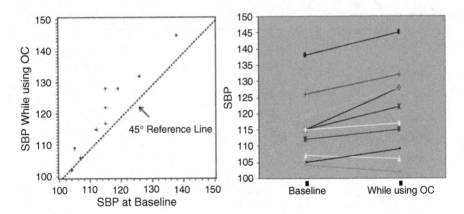

Fig. 3.6 Illustration of paired continuous outcomes data visual display

Subject	Baseline SBP	Follow up SBP	Difference (d_i) of the repeated measures
1	115	128	13
2	112	115	3
3	107	106	-1
4	119	128	9
5	115	122	7
6	138	145	7
7	126	132	6
8	105	109	4
9	104	102	-2
10	115	117	2
Mean	115.60	120.40	4.80
SD	10.31	13.22	4.57
SE	3.26	4.18	1.44

Note: This single column data can be used for testing if the population mean difference is zero by "one-sample" t-test

Fig. 3.7 Illustration of calculated paired differences can be analyzed by a one-sample *t*-test

hypotheses. By letting δ denote $\mu_2 - \mu_1$, the null and alternative hypotheses are rewritten as H_0: $\delta = 0$ and H_1: $\delta \neq 0$. The observed estimate of δ is the sample mean of ten changes in SBP between the baseline and follow-up d is 4.80, and the null value is 0. The $SE(d - \delta) = SE(d)$ is directly estimated from the ten within-subject longitudinal changes. The resulting test statistic is the same as that of the one-sample t-test as the within-subject change is treated as the unit of analysis, which is depicted by Figs. 3.7 and 3.8. The test statistic $t = (d - \delta)/ SE(d - \delta) = d/SE(d)$ follows the *t*-distribution with $df = n \ of \ pairs - 1 = 10{-}1 = 9$.

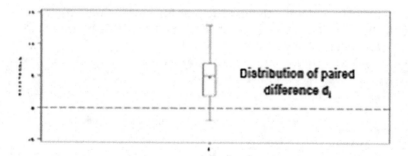

Fig. 3.8 Box-and-whisker plot applied to describe the distribution of differences calculated from pairs of continuous outcomes

The resulting t = (4.8 - 0) / 1.44 = 3.324 and p-value is 0.0089, which indicates that the mean change of 4.8 was significant at 5 % significance level.

The paired samples t-test, as the raw data are reduced into the pair-wise within-subject differences, is the same as the one-sample t-test, df is the number of unique individuals – 1.

A common misapplication of the t-test to the paired data is to apply the independent samples t-test. As illustrated below, such an erroneous application would mislead the study investigation. If the equal population variance independent samples t-test (see Table 3.2 in Sect. 3.1.2) had been applied to the above example, then the test statistic's denominator, $SE(\bar{x}_2 - \bar{x}_1)$, where $\bar{x}_1$ and $\bar{x}_2$ are the baseline and follow-up mean SBPs, is to apply $\sqrt{(s^2_1/n + s^2_2/n)} = \sqrt{(2s^2_p/n)}$, where $s^2_p = [s^2_1/(n_1-1) + s^2_2/(n_1-1)/(n_1-1 + n_1-1)]$, $n_1=n_2=10$, $s^2_1 = 10.31^2$, and $s^2_2 = 13.22^2$. The calculated value of this standard error is 5.3028. Then the test statistic $t = (4.8 - 0)/5.3028 = 0.91$ with $df = 18$. The p-value is 0.3773, which is contradictory to the result from the paired sample t-test.

3.3   Use of Excel for t-Tests

The one-sample, independent samples, and paired samples t-tests can easily be carried out using Excel (Figs. 3.9, 3.10, and 3.11).

3.4   Study Questions

1. Explain the idea of "*Observed~Expected~Standard Error*" formulation of the test statistic t of the independent samples t-test.
2. Can the paired samples t-test be conceived as a one-sample t-test? Why?

Use of Excel to perform a **diagnostic test for heteroskedasticity**
before choosing the proper independent samples t-tests between the
equal- versus unequal variance versions

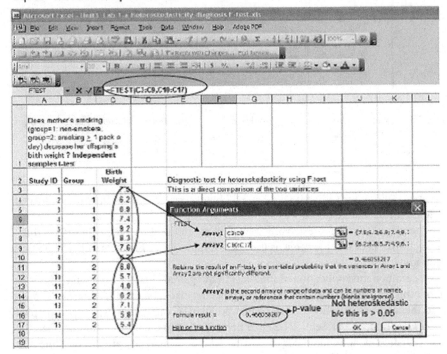

Fig. 3.9 Use of excel function FTEST for testing equality of two variances

3. What is the idea behind to decrease the degrees of freedom for the independent
   samples *t*-test when the variances of the two populations are not equal?
4. Please criticize the following awkward sentences:

   "These data showed that the two groups were significantly different (p<0.05)."
   "These data showed that the two group means were significantly different."
   "The calculated *p*-value was less than 0.05 thus we rejected the null
   hypothesis."

Use of Excel to perform **Independent Samples t-test**

Independent t-test, i.e., Two Sample Unpaired T-test using Excel

Please see how the data are entered into the spread sheet; and see the
array 1 and array 2, and the options given to TTEST function.

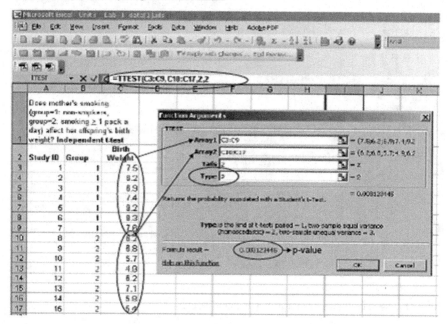

Fig. 3.10 Use of excel function for independent samples *t*-tests

Use of Excel to perform **Paired Samples t-test**

Paired t-test

Please see how the data are entered into the spread sheet; and see the
array 1 and array 2, and the options given to TTEST function.

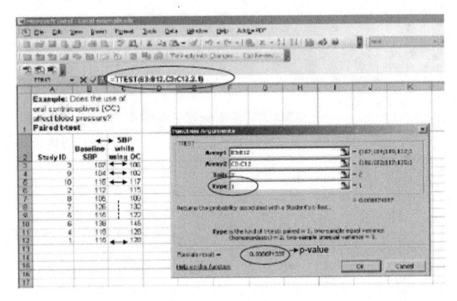

Fig. 3.11   Use of excel function for paired samples *t*-test

Bibliography

Dawson B, Trapp RG (1994) Basic & clinical biostatistics, 4th edn. Appleton & Lange, Norwalk
Glantz SA (2005) Primer of biostatistics, 6th edn. McGraw Hill Professional, New York
Pagano M, Gauvreau K (1993) Principles of biostatistics. Duxbury Press, Belmont
Rosner B (2010) Fundamentals of biostatistics, 7th edn. Cengage Learnings, Boston
Snecdecor GW, Cochran WG (1991) Statistical methods, 8th edn. Wiley-Blackwell, Malden
Zar JH (2010) Biostatistical analysis, 5th edn. Prentice-Hall/Pearson, Upper Saddle River

Chapter 4
Inference Using Analysis of Variance for Comparing Multiple Means

This chapter discusses single-factor analysis of variance (ANOVA) which is mainly applied to compare three or more independent means. The words "single factor" refer to that the means are compared across levels of a "single" classification variable (i.e., classification of means by a single categorical variable). The classification variable is called independent variable or factor (thus, the method is also called single-factor ANOVA) and the outcome variable of which the means are compared is called dependent variable. This method requires certain assumptions: (1) the dependent variable values are the observations sampled from a normal distribution and (2) the population variances are equal (homoscedasticity) across the levels of the independent variable (Fig. 4.1).

Having mentioned that ANOVA is mainly applied to compare three or more means, is it obvious why the variance is analyzed in order to compare the means? The ANOVA is a two-step procedure. The first step is to measure two partitioned pieces of outcome data variations due to two sources of variations, of which the first piece is the variation of the outcome variable explained by the groups being compared and the second is the unexplained residual (error) variation. The next step is to utilize these two data variations to carry out the hypothesis testing for comparing the means. These data variations are measured by means of sums of squares (see Sect. 1.3.4).

4.1 Sums of Squares and Variances

In Fig. 4.2, three groups of sample data that are clearly separated (for illustrative purpose) by the underlying group effects are illustrated, and the symmetrically scattered outcomes around their group means reveal the random sampling error. ANOVA is to examine whether or not the group effect depicted by the distances among the three group means can separate the group-wise data cluster in the presence of the ransom sampling error. The group effect (i.e., signal) and the random sampling error (i.e., noise) are measured by two kinds of sums of squares first and then transformed into kinds of average sum of squares (so-called mean squares).

H. Lee, *Foundations of Applied Statistical Methods*, DOI 10.1007/978-3-319-02402-8_4,
© Springer International Publishing Switzerland 2014

Fig. 4.1 Illustration of
density curves of three
continuous outcomes with
unequal means and equal
variances

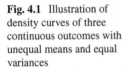
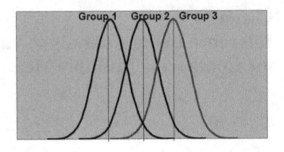

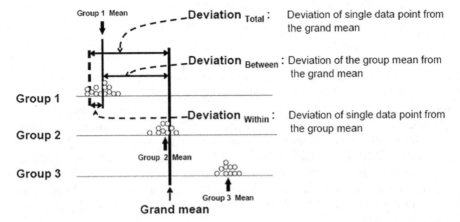

Fig. 4.2 Illustration of three kinds of deviations arising from comparing three independent means

Figure 4.3 demonstrates the concepts of derivations and these sums of squares
(*SS*) that are the underpinnings of ANOVA. For instance, the first observed outcome
value 5 (Sample Number 1 in Group 1) is conceived as a value deviated by −15 from
the single grand mean of 20; this outcome is also conceived as a value deviated by
−5 from its group mean 10 wherein this group mean is deviated by −10 from the
grand mean 20. It is obvious that the three corresponding squared deviations are
$(-15)^2 = 225$, $(-5)^2 = 25$, and $(-10)^2 = 100$. Repeating the same calculation over every
observation within each group and cumulating the resulted individual squared deviations into the group sum totals, and then summing the group sum totals over the all
three groups finally produces three kinds of sums of squares. These three sums of
squares are called total-, between-, and within-sum of squares and the resulting
values are 950, 800, and 150, respectively. Intuitively, the total sum of squares of
950 is partitioned into between-group sum of squares of 800 and within-group sum
of squares of 150.

Dividing a sum of squares by a divisor (i.e., degrees of freedom, see Sect. 2.2.3) is a
kind of variance. In ANOVA, two such variances are compared, and these are the variance due to the group difference and the variance due to the sampling error (i.e., unexplained residual variance by the systematic group difference). In order to distinguish the
meaning of the ordinary variance, these variances being obtained in ANOVA are termed

Sum of Squares in Single Factor ANOVA

Sample Number	Group	Observed Outcome Value	Deviation of Each Single Data Point from Grand Mean			Squared Deviation of Each Single Data Point from Grand Mean	Squared Deviation of Each Group Mean from Grand Mean	Squared Deviation of Each Single Data Point from Group Mean
			Dev. Single from Grand	Dev. Group from Grand	Dev. Single from Group			
1	1	5	-15 =	-10 +	-5	225	100	25
2	1	10	-10 =	-10 +	0	100	100	0
3	1	10	-10 =	-10 +	0	100	100	0
4	1	15	-5 =	-10 +	5	25	100	25
		Group 1 Mean = 10				Sub total =450	Sub total =400	Sub total =50
5	2	15	-5 =	0 +	-5	25	0	25
6	2	20	0 =	0 +	0	0	0	0
7	2	20	0 =	0 +	0	0	0	0
8	2	25	5 =	0 +	5	25	0	25
		Group 2 Mean = 20				Sub total =50	Sub total =0	Sub total =50
9	3	25	5 =	10 +	-5	25	100	25
10	3	30	10 =	10 +	0	100	100	0
11	3	30	10 =	10 +	0	100	100	0
12	3	35	15 =	10 +	5	225	100	25
		Group 3 Mean = 30				Sub total =450	Sub total =400	Sub total =50
		Grand Mean = 20				SS Total = 950	Between 800	SS Within 150

SS Total = Between + SS Within

Fig. 4.3 Formulae-less numerical illustration of sum of squares in single-factor ANOVA

mean squares (denoted by MS). The two major mean squares in the single-factor ANOVA are the between-group mean square ($MS_{between}$) and the within-group mean square (MS_{within}). $MS_{between}$ is the sum of squared deviations from the grand mean for all data values divided by its divisor for which the divisor is one less than the number of unique deviations of the group means from the referenced overall grand mean. Note that as demonstrated in Fig. 4.3, there are only three unique deviations of the group means from the grand mean, and the $MS_{between}$ becomes $(400+0+400)/(3-1)=800/2=400$. MS_{within} is $50+50+50/[$ (number of unique deviations of the individual data points from the Group 1 mean $-1)+$ (number of unique deviations of the individual data points from the Group 2 mean $-1)+$ (number of unique deviations of the individual data points from the Group 3 mean $-1)]=150/[(4-1)+(4-1)+(4-1)]=150/9=16.67)$.

4.2   F-Test

After the between- and within-group mean squares are obtained, the inference to compare means is performed. The null and alternative hypotheses are H_0: $\mu_1 = \mu_2 = \mu_3$, ..., μ_k (all means are equal) and H_1: at least one mean is different (not all means are equal), respectively. The test statistic is derived under the assumption that the data are drawn from normally distributed populations and the population variances are

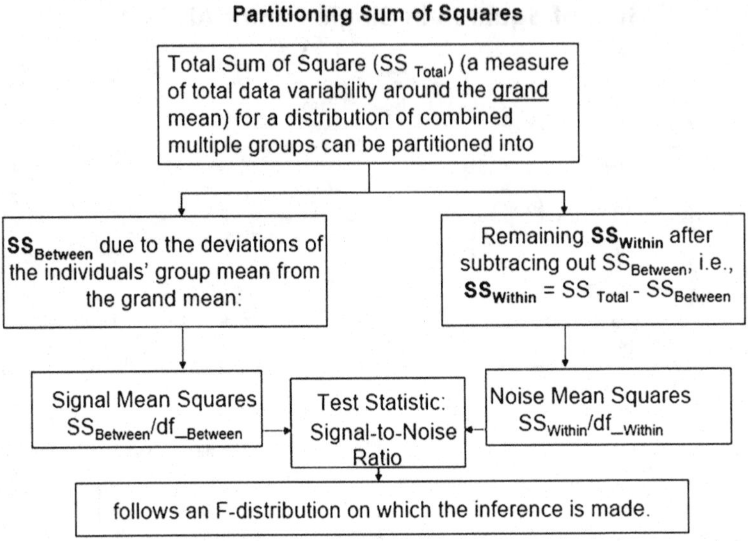

Partitioning Sum of Squares

Total Sum of Square (SS $_{Total}$) (a measure of total data variability around the <u>grand</u> mean) for a distribution of combined multiple groups can be partitioned into

SS$_{Between}$ due to the deviations of the individuals' group mean from the grand mean:

Remaining SS$_{Within}$ after subtracing out SS$_{Between}$, i.e., SS$_{Within}$ = SS $_{Total}$ - SS$_{Between}$

Signal Mean Squares SS$_{Between}$/df$_{\_Between}$

Test Statistic: Signal-to-Noise Ratio

Noise Mean Squares SS$_{Within}$/df$_{\_Within}$

follows an F-distribution on which the inference is made.

Fig. 4.4 Partitioning sum of squares for single-factor ANOVA

equal across the groups. Unlike the t-tests, the test statistic of this test is not derived from the "triplet" idea (see Sects. 2.2.4.5 and 3.1). Instead, the ratio of the two mean squares (see Sect. 4.1) is used as the test statistic. By letting F denote this ratio, $F = MS_{between}/MS_{within}$ is the signal (of the between-group difference)-to-noise (random sampling error) ratio test statistic. Under the null hypothesis, this test statistic follows an F-distribution which is characterized by two degrees of freedom, $df_{between}$ and df_{within}. Each df is the divisor that is used for calculating the mean squares and each divisor is one less than the number of unique squared deviations from the referenced mean that are summed into the SS calculations.

In the case of Fig. 4.4 example, $F = 400/16.67 = 23.99$ is a particular value of the F-distribution with $df_{between} = 2$ and $df_{within} = 9$. The rejection region for this test statistic is depicted in Fig. 4.5 wherein the presented curve represents the density function of the sampling distribution F with the two required degrees of freedom 2 and 9, respectively. Evidently, such a large value 23.99 fell into the rejection region (i.e., $F > 4.275$); thus these data showed the evidence to reject H_0 at a 5 % significance level.

Area above 4,257 is 0.05, thus $F > 4.257$ is the rejection region of F value for the single-factor ANOVA F-test at 5 % significance level to compare three means with four observations in each group.

Example 4.1

A cross-sectional study design is applied in order to examine if mother's smoking affected offspring's birth weight. The null and alternative hypotheses for the inference are H_0: $\mu_1 = \mu_2 = \mu_3 = \mu_4$ (all four means are equal) and H_1: at least one mean is different (not all means are equal), respectively.

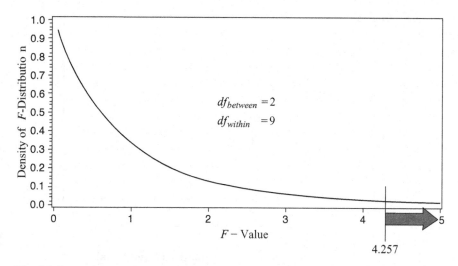

Fig. 4.5 Determination of the rejection region of the F-distribution for an ANOVA F-test for comparing three means using data set illustrated in Fig. 4.4

Table 4.1 ANOVA source table

Source of variation	SS	df	MS	F	p-Value
Between group	11.74	3	3.91	4.20	0.017
Within group	21.28	23	0.93		
Total	33.02	26			

The following data are birth weights (lb) of 27 newborns classified by their maternal smoking status (i.e., one-way classification). The data normality is assumed.

Group 1—Mother is a nonsmoker (n=7): 7.5 6.2 6.9 7.4 9.2 8.3 7.6
Group 2—Mother is an ex-smoker (n=5): 5.8 7.3 8.2 7.1 7.8
Group 3—Mother smokes <1 pack/day (n=7): 5.9 6.2 5.8 4.7 8.3 7.2 6.2
Group 4—Mother smokes ≥ 1 pack/day (n=8): 6.2 6.8 5.7 4.9 6.2 7.1 5.8 5.4

The means and standard deviations are obtained as the descriptive summary statistics. Besides these descriptive statistics, a summary table (so-called ANOVA table) is traditionally to present the sum of square and mean square for each source of variation as well as the test statistic F and its p-value (see Table 4.1).

Computation of the sums of squares and mean squares can be done either by a computer package program or manually. As this chapter does not offer the directly usable computational formulae, this illustration is made in order solely to walk you through the essential computations of the variance partitioning and the derivation of the test statistic.

The first quantity to calculate is how much the group means are deviated from the grand mean, where the grand mean, $\bar{x}_G$, is the weighted average of the four means where the weights are the group sample sizes, i.e., $\bar{x}_G = (7 \times 7.59 + 5 \times 7.24 + 7 \times 6.33 + 8 \times 6.01)/27 = 6.73$. $SS_{between}$ is the summation of sum of seven of squared unique

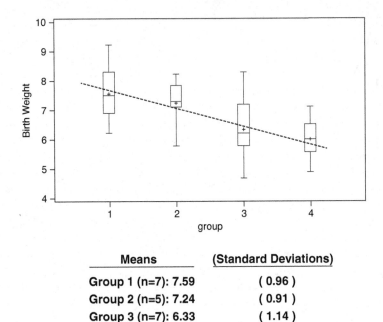

Means	(Standard Deviations)
Group 1 (n=7): 7.59	(0.96)
Group 2 (n=5): 7.24	(0.91)
Group 3 (n=7): 6.33	(1.14)
Group 4 (n=8): 6.01	(0.72)

Fig. 4.6 Box-and-whisker plot of four distributions of which their means are compared by single-factor ANOVA F-test

Group 1 sample mean's deviation from the grand mean, i.e., $7 \times (\bar{x}_1 - \bar{x}_G)^2$, summation of sum of five of such squared value from Group 2, i.e., $5 \times (\bar{x}_2 - \bar{x}_G)^2$, $7 \times (\bar{x}_3 - \bar{x}_G)^2$ from Group 3, and $8 \times (\bar{x}_4 - \bar{x}_G)^2$ from Group 4, which is $7 \times (7.59 - 6.73)^2 + 5 \times (7.24 - 6.73)^2 + 7 \times (6.33 - 6.73)^2 + 8 \times (6.01 - 6.73)^2 = 11.74$. SS_{within} is the summation of 4 within-group sum of squares, of which each within-group sum of square is obtainable from the already calculated within-group standard deviation. Because s_k^2 is $(n_k - 1)/(n_k - 1)$, where $k = 1, 2, 3,$ and 4 indicating the group, SS_{within} for group $k = s_k^2 \times (n_k - 1)$. Therefore, $SS_{within}/(n_k - 1)$ from all four groups $= (7 - 1) \times 0.96^2 + (5 - 1) \times 0.91^2 + (7 - 1) \times 1.14^2 + (8 - 1) \times 0.72^2 = 21.28$. Finally, $F = MS_{between} / MS_{within} = [11.74/(4 - 1)]/[21.28/(7-1)+(5-1)+(7-1)+(8-1)] = (11.74/3)/(21.28/23) = 3.91 / 0.93 = 4.20$. Finally, the p-value was directly evaluated by using Excel (not by determining the critical region and seeing if the observed F value fell into the critical region), i.e., $p = \text{FDIST} (4.20, df_{between} = 3, df_{within} = 23) = 0.017$. Figure 4.7 is the graphical demonstration for this calculation wherein the density function of an F-distribution is characterized by the two required degrees of freedom, and 3 and 23 appeared differently from the one with degrees of freedom 2 and 9 (Fig. 4.5). Note that the shape of density curve of an F-distribution is characterized by the degrees of freedom (i.e., not all F-distributions look similar).

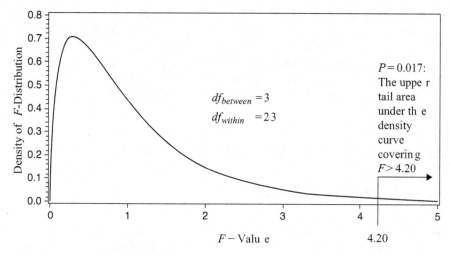

Fig. 4.7 *p*-Value calculation of the *F*-statistic obtained from an ANOVA *F*-test comparing three means using data set illustrated in Fig. 4.6

Although the *p*-value was directly calculated in this example, the significance can also be determined by checking if the test statistic fell into the critical region. The critical region of this test is *F > 3.03*, which is found from the critical value table of *F*-distribution at 5 % significance level with the between- and within-group degrees of freedom of 3 and 23.

The suggestive format of the summary sentence is either "These data showed that at least one age group's mean birth weight is significantly different from the means of the other age groups (*p* = 0.017)." or "These data showed that at least one age group's mean birth weight is significantly different from the means of the other age groups at 5 % significance level."

4.3   Multiple Comparisons and Increased Type-1 Error

Suppose H_0: $\mu_1 = \mu_2 = \mu_3 = \mu_4$ in favor of H_1: at least one mean differs from the others was rejected by a one-way ANOVA *F*-test. It remains ambiguous which specific means differed until all possible pair-wise tests (6 independent samples *t*-test can be performed in this case) comparing two groups at a time. In doing so, the increased number of tests increases the potential Type-1 error. In order to protect from such an increased chance of committing Type-1 error, a stringent criterion (i.e., modified significance level) for these tests need to be adopted. One of such options is to lower the significance level of each test by dividing it by the number of comparisons (Bonferroni's correction, i.e., adjusted $\alpha = 0.05/6 = 0.0083$, or to inflate the computed *p*-value by multiplying it by the number of comparisons, i.e., inflated *p*-value = 6 × observed *p*-value). However, this tends to be too conservative as the number of tests increases. Many *"not-too-conservative but powerful"* tests have been invented. Least Significance Difference (LSD), Highly Significant Difference (HSD), Student–Newman–Keuls (SNK), and Duncan's Multiple Range Test procedures are popularized procedures applying pair-wise multiple tests for comparing means, and Dunnett's procedure is a procedure to compare ordered groups with a baseline group using modified critical values of the test statistic.

4.4 Beyond Single-Factor ANOVA

4.4.1 Multi-factor ANOVA

As the number of categorical independent variables increase and the outcomes are classified by these independent variables, the ANOVA F-tests will involve the partitioning of the total variance into the between-group variances due to the effects of these individual independent variables, the between-group variances due to the interactions of two or more independent variables, and the remaining variance that is not explained by those sources of variations that are already taken into account. The testing procedure for comparing subgroup means (e.g., difference of the means among the levels of the first independent variable, that among the levels of second independent variable, and that among the levels arising from the interaction of the first and second independent variables) is F-test, of which the test statistic's numerator is the mean square due to the between-group effect of interest and the denominator is the unexplained error mean square. With a firm understanding of the single-factor ANOVA, it becomes a trial technique to extend the method to the multi-factor ANOVA. However, it would be worth addressing the definition and interpretation of the interaction, and the repeated measures ANOVA as a special case of two-factor ANOVA to which the following two sections are devoted.

4.4.2 Interaction

The following example focuses onto illustrating the definition of interaction as well as the marginal means, main effects, and simple means arising in the two-factor ANOVA. The example is self-explanatory that does not necessitate the verbal definitions.

Example 4.2

A study of abdominal fat reduction (measured in % reduction) after 8-week programs of exercise alone or diet + exercise conducted involving two age groups of age <50 years and age ≥50 years. Sample size of each subgroup was 2,000. Let's assume that every observed difference was statistically significant.

Q1. Please show: (a) marginal means; (b) main effects; and (c) simple effects.

(a) Marginal means: Marginal mean of Program $1 = (5+3)/2 \rightarrow 4$ %; marginal mean of Program $2 = (8+4)/2 \rightarrow 6$ % regardless of the age; marginal mean of Age < 50 is $(5+8)/2 \rightarrow 6.5$ %, and marginal mean of age $>=50$ is $(3+4)/2 \rightarrow 3.5$ % regardless of the program type.

(b) Main effects (effects towards the healthier outcome): Program main effect (Marginal mean of Program 2 – Marginal mean of Program $1 = (8+4)/2$ - $(5+3)/2 = 6 - 4 \rightarrow 2$ %, meaning that Program 1 reduced a 2 % greater fat reduction in all ages; Age main effect (Mean of Age < 50 - Mean of Age $>=50) = (5+8)/2$ $- (3+4)/2 = 6.5 - 3.5 \rightarrow 3$ %, meaning the younger age group showed a greater reduction on average regardless of the program.

(c) Simple effects: The four specific means by themselves simply exhibit the age- and program-specific subgroup mean outcomes and do not directly describe the "effects (i.e., mean differences)." Simple effect is the size of mean difference within each group. Program 2 vs. 1 simple effect within Age <50 is 3 % (i.e., 8 $- 5 \rightarrow 3$ %); Program 2 vs. 1 simple effect within Age ≥ 50 is 1 % (i.e., 4 – $3 \rightarrow 1$ %); also Age <50 vs. ≥ 50 simple effect within Program 1 is 2 %, and that of Program 2 is 4 %.

Q2. Was there an interaction? If so, please describe the observed phenomenon.

There was an interaction in that the younger age group's Program 2 vs. Program 1 effect in mean reduction was greater than that of the older age group. The younger age group showed three times better performance (i.e., 8 $-$ 5 $\rightarrow$ 3 % reduction in the younger age group by adding diet to the exercise vs. 4–3 $\rightarrow$ 1 % reduction in the older age group by adding diet to the exercise). Yes, there was an interaction (i.e., age interacted with the programs). Note that the word "interaction" is a phenomenon, and its quantitative is the difference in simple effects of the two age groups (i.e., [8–5 $\rightarrow$ 3 % in age < 50] – [4–3 $\rightarrow$ 1 % in Age ≥ 50] = 2 %). If both age groups had shown the same mean fat reduction differences between the two programs we would have pronounced that there was no interaction (Table 4.2).

Table 4.2   Means of % fat reduction by age group and program

	Program 1: exercise alone	Program 2: exercise and diet
Age <50	n=2,000	n=2,000
	Mean reduction=5 %	Mean reduction=8 %
Age ≥50	n=2,000	n=2,000
	Mean reduction=3 %	Mean reduction=4 %

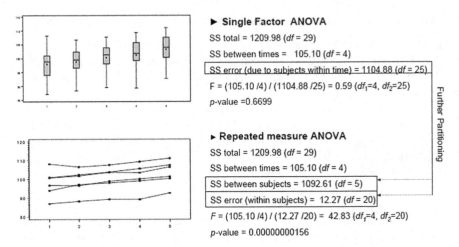

Fig. 4.8 Illustration of improved result by repeated measures ANOVA compared to single-factor ANOVA

4.4.3   Repeated Measures ANOVA

The importance of choosing the appropriate method to take into account the source of variation arising from the study design and experiment cannot be overemphasized. The paired samples t-test is applied to compare two related means (e.g., pre- to post-mean difference) because the independent samples t-test does not take into account the related individual paired measures. Many approaches as a means to the companion to the paired samples t-test are available for comparing more than two related means. Depending on the particular patterns of the within-subject correlation among more than two repeated measures, there are various technical options to deal with the situations. The repeated measures ANOVA is one of such options and its idea is illustrated in Fig. 4.8. This illustrated data analysis was to study whether or not the means of the repeatedly measured outcomes changed over time, i.e., H_0: $\mu_1 = \mu_2 = \mu_3 = \mu_4 = \mu_5$ vs. H_1: not all five means are equal (i.e., at least one mean at a particular time is different from the rest), by measuring the longitudinal (i.e., those five serial outcomes are related within a subject) outcomes from six (n=6) individual subjects. The first part of the illustration is a result from applying the single-factor ANOVA F-test, which was not appropriate because it did not take into account the repeated measurements. Let us discuss which explainable source of variation could have been taken into account if the analysis had been done by an appropriate method. The box-and-whisker plot showed a gradually increasing pattern of the means over time, but the single-factor ANOVA F-test's p-value was 0.6699 (i.e., not significant at 5 % alpha level). Keeping in mind that these data are repeated measures, the individual subject-specific unique patterns (i.e., trajectory over time) and their difference between the subjects could be a new explainable source of outcome variation. As depicted by the second plot (so-called spaghetti plot) the visualized six individual trajectories describe the data variation differently than what was possible solely by the box-and-whisker plot. What can be pointed out by this spaghetti plot is that there was a common trend of increasing pattern among the subjects and a non-ignorable portion of the overall outcome spread-out (i.e., total variance) was clearly due to the initial baseline variation among the subjects (i.e., the trajectories did not cross over very much). For this reason, it is reasonable to add the between-subjects variation as a newly explainable source of data variation. As shown in the two ANOVA tables, SS *between subjects* in the repeated measures ANOVA summary was partitioned out from the previous SS *error* (between- and within-subjects had been combined) of the single-factor ANOVA (i.e., $1104.88 \rightarrow 1092.61 + 12.27$). Finally, the smaller portion that has not been still unexplained by time and between-subject variability sources remained as SS *error* (only within-subjects), thus the p-value of the repeated measures ANOVA F-test for the time effect resulted much smaller than that of the single-factor ANOVA F-test. Note that this approach is indeed the same as to apply a two-factor ANOVA in which the between-subject effect is considered the second factor. This illustration skipped the detailed calculation involved in the analysis because it is unnecessarily laborious without using computers. The objective of this illustration was to focus mainly onto the rationale of taking into account the repeated measures and its impact to improve the result and interpretation.

4.4.4 Use of Excel for ANOVA

Excel offers the ANOVA procedure for single-factor, two-factor, and repeated measures ANOVA. The features allow only the data sets of which the group sample sizes are equal. However, such data sets can still be handled by Excel via regression analysis with dummy variable (see Chap. 5).

4.5 Study Questions

1. Using Excel sheet, please carry out the computation of sums of squares for the one-way ANOVA and F-test (H_0: H_0: $\mu_1 = \mu_2 = \mu_3$) of these data (similar demonstration is available in Fig. 4.3):

   Sample data from Group 1: 1, 2, 3, 4, 5
   Sample data from Group 2: 4, 5, 6
   Sample data from Group 3: 6, 7, 8

2. Give these descriptive statistics, please figure out what are the $SS_{between}$ and SS_{within} for the one-way ANOVA

   Group 1: $n = 9$, mean $= 10$, variance $= 36$
   Group 2: $n = 10$, mean $= 15$, variance $= 36$
   Group 3: $n = 11$, mean $= 20$, variance $= 36$

3. If the independent samples t-test is applied to compare two means and the population variances are equal, can the one-way ANOVA be applied to this inference? If so, will the p-value from the applied one-way ANOVA be the same as that resulted from the independent samples t-test?

Bibliography

Cox DR, Snell EJ (1981) Applied statistics: principles and examples. Chapman and Hall, New York
Glantz SA (2005) Primer of biostatistics, 6th edn. McGraw Hill Professional, New York
Pagano M, Gauvreau K (1993) Principles of biostatistics. Duxbury Press, Belmont, CA
Rosner B (2010) Fundamentals of biostatistics, 7th edn. Cengage Learnings Inc., Independence, KY
Scheffé H (1999) The analysis of variance. Wiley, New York
Winer BJ (1971) Statistical principles in experimental design, 2nd edn. McGraw-Hill, New York

Chapter 5
Linear Correlation and Regression

In Chap. 1, Pearson's correlation coefficient as a means to describe a linear association between two continuous measures was introduced. In this chapter, the inference of the correlation coefficient using sample data will be discussed first, and then the discussion will extend to a related method and its inference to examine a linear association of the continuous and binary outcomes with one or more variables using sample data.

5.1 Inference of a Single Pearson's Correlation Coefficient

A linear association measured by the Pearson's correlation coefficient between two continuous measures obtained from a sample, r, requires an inference. The two forms of inferences are hypothesis testing and interval estimation (i.e., construction of the confidence interval). Testing hypothesis is to state the null and alternative hypotheses, compute the test statistic, and determine if it is significant. Let us discuss the hypothesis testing first. The null hypothesis is that there is no linear association between two continuous outcomes (i.e., H_0: $\rho=0$), and the alternative hypothesis is either a nondirectional alternative hypothesis (i.e., H_1: $\rho \neq 0$) or a directional alternative hypothesis (i.e., H_1: $\rho>0$, or H_1: $\rho<0$), depending on the researcher's objective. For such an inference we need a test statistic. A typical test statistic involves an arithmetic transformation of the sample correlation coefficient r because the sampling distribution of r is not approximately normal even when the sample size becomes large (i.e., the CLT is not applicable for the sample correlation coefficient). Nonetheless, it is noted that the sampling distribution of the transformation $z = \frac{1}{2}[ln(1+r) - ln(1-r)]$ will follow $N(0, 1/\sqrt{(n-3)})$ under the null hypothesis as the number of observed data pairs, n, becomes sufficiently large. The idea of "*Observed Estimate ~ Null Value ~ SE* triplet (see Sect. 2.2.4.2)" is then applied to derive the test statistic. Instead of directly plugging in the observed sample correlation r, the above z transformation is substituted for the *observed estimate*,

H. Lee, *Foundations of Applied Statistical Methods*, DOI 10.1007/978-3-319-02402-8_5,
© Springer International Publishing Switzerland 2014

Table 5.1 Smallest absolute values of sample correlations that are significantly different from 0 by nondirectional t-test

| $df=n$ of pairs–2 | Level of significance of a one-sample nondirectional t-test (H_0: $\rho=0$ versus H_1: $\rho\neq0$) | | |
	10 %	5 %	1 %
3	0.805	0.878	0.959
10	0.497	0.576	0.708
15	0.412	0.482	0.606
20	0.360	0.423	0.537
25	0.323	0.381	0.487
30	0.296	0.381	0.449

i.e., $z = \{0.5 \cdot [ln(1+r) - ln(1-r)] - 0\}/\sqrt{(n-3)}$, so that the sampling distribution of this resulting test statistic z can follow the standard normal distribution.

For small sample size, this test statistic can be resorted to t-distribution (i.e., one-sample t-test). The following table lists the minimum values of the sample correlation coefficients that would become statistically significant by a nondirectional t-test of which H_0: $\rho=0$ and H_1: $\rho\neq0$ for various sample sizes (Table 5.1).

The interval estimation can also be made by using this z-statistic. The lower and upper 95 % confidence limits of the population correlation coefficient can be obtained in two steps, of which the first step is to find the lower and upper 95 % confidence limits (i.e., 2.5th and 97.5th percentiles of the sampling distribution) of z, then equating these two limits to the expression $\{0.5 [ln(1+ \rho) - ln(1- \rho)] - 0\}/\sqrt{(n-3)}$, then finally solving them for ρ.

5.1.1   Q & A Discussion

Question: In correlation analyses, to what extent should we look at the r-value and the p-value? For instance, is $r=0.7$ ($p<0.05$), "stronger" than $r=0.5$ ($p<0.001$)? Is $r=0.1$ a poor correlation even if $p<0.001$? Is $r=0.8$ a good correlation even if $p>0.1$?

Answer: The magnitude of r and its p-value cannot be interpreted universally. The cross comparison of the magnitudes of r's is only meaningful within one data set where all the r's are obtained from the same sample size. Don't compare apples with oranges.

5.2   Linear Regression Model with One Independent Variable: Simple Regression Model

A statistical model usually appears as a mathematical description (often involves mathematical expression, i.e., equations, etc.) of how individual datum is determined with uncertainty (i.e., random sampling error). Linear regression model with one independent variable describes how a numeric (normally distributed) outcome (i.e., dependent) variable is determined by one independent nonrandom variable and a random error. More specifically, it appears as an equation where the left-hand side is the outcome variable and the right-hand side consists of two parts of which the first part articulates the nonrandom common rule and the second does the random error (i.e., individuals' deviations from the nonrandom common rule).

The following is a typical expression of the ith observed outcome y_i described by the linear regression model with one independent variable:

$$y_i = \underset{\underset{\text{Common rule}}{\uparrow}}{\beta_0 + \beta_1 X_i +} \quad \underset{\underset{\text{Random phenomenon}}{\uparrow}}{\varepsilon_i},$$

where ε_i, for individual i, is a random error term that follows a normal distribution with mean$=0$ and variance$=\sigma^2$. The ith observed outcome y_i is expressed by the common value that is the same as the value for all other observations as long as the value of the independent variable is given to a certain value plus the random deviation from the common value. The regression refers to the rule, how this common value of the dependent variable is determined given a certain value of the independent variable. This model is called a *simple linear* regression model. It is called *simple* because there is only one independent variable and called *linear* because the common rule is expressed by a linear function of the independent variable. As discussed later in this chapter, a *multiple* (as opposed to simple) linear regression model is a linear model that includes more than one independent variable, e.g., $y_i = \beta_0 + \beta_1 x_1 + \beta_2 x_2 + \ldots + \varepsilon_i$.

The simple regression model can have its variants, and the following is such an example:

$$y_i = \beta_0 + \beta_1 X^2_i + \varepsilon_i,$$

where ε_i, for individual i, is a random error term that follows a normal distribution with mean$=0$ and variance$=\sigma^2$. First, how many independent variables are there? Only one, so the *simple* part makes sense. Having x^2 in the model as the independent variable does not mean this is a nonlinear model. Let's note that the word *linear* means that the nonrandom common rule, $\beta_0 + \beta_1 x^2_i$, is linearly determined by a given value of the independent variable (i.e., the rate of linear change is β_1 for a unit change of x^2, and the amount $\beta_1 x^2_i$ determined by a particular value of x^2 is additive to β_0). To make it clearer, one can rename x^2 to a new name z, i.e., $y_i = \beta_0 + \beta_1 z_i + \varepsilon_i$.

5.3   Simple Linear Regression Analysis

Regression analysis is to seek the best common rule equation that determines the mean value of the outcome variable given a certain value of the independent variable. The widely used computational procedure is the least squares method.

Fig. 5.1 Illustration of the least squares method to estimate linear regression equation

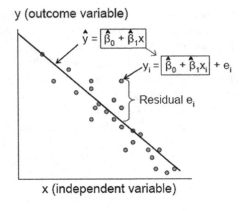

In Fig. 5.1, the drawn line is the estimated regression line determined by the least squares method. Residual e_i is the difference between the observed y_i and the predicted value $\hat{y}_i$ via the estimated sample regression line. Note that the residual e_i is not the same random error term ε_i introduced in the model specification in that the term ε_i specified is the difference between the observed and the true population regression line. The least squares method is to estimate the intercept and slope of the regression line that minimize sum of squared residuals, e_i^2. The resulting estimated line is indeed the whole collection of the predicted means of the outcome variable y given the values of the independent variable x when the normality assumption of the ε_i error term's distribution is true. Computer programs (even Excel software has the feature) are widely available for estimating each regression equation parameter (i.e., intercept β_0, and slope β_1) and the standard error of each estimated regression parameter, and for providing the test statistic of the hypothesis testing whether or not each of the population coefficient is different from zero, as well as the 95 % confidence interval of each regression parameter.

A goodness of fit for the estimated simple linear regression equation is measured by r^2. This metric is the same as the squared value of the sample linear correlation coefficient computed from the observed y and x pairs. It is also the same as the proportion of the explained variation of the dependent variable by the estimated regression equation. The possible range is from 0 (0 % is explained) to 1 (100 % is explained). The r^2 is 1 – (sum of squares of the residuals/sum of squares deviations of the observed outcome values from the overall mean of the outcome values). Figure 5.2 illustrates the concept of r^2 and demonstrates the computational details. The first plot depicts the r^2 in the absence of a fitted regression equation for which the horizontal line represents the mean of y irrespective of the values of independent variable. The second plot depicts the r^2 of the fitted regression equation. It is also noted that r^2 is the squared value of the correlation coefficient between y and $\hat{y}$, and it is also the same as the squared value of the correlation coefficient between y and x. This can be shown algebraically and numerically.

Let's use an example of a simple linear regression equation estimated from an analysis, $y = 64.30 + 1.39 \cdot x$, where y denotes systolic blood pressure (SBP) and x

Get sum of sq. of deviations of y values from the mean before fitting a regression equation

Get sum of sq. of deviations of the y values from the predicted $\hat{y}$ by x

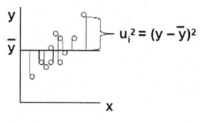

$$u_i^2 = (y - \bar{y})^2$$

$$e_i^2 = (y - \hat{y})^2$$

$$\hat{y} = \hat{\beta}_0 + \hat{\beta}_1 x$$

$$r^2 = 1 - (\Sigma e_i^2) / (\Sigma u_i^2)$$

Estiamted Regression equation $\hat{y} = 4.73 + 0.43 \cdot x$ (Computer provided result)

y	x	$\bar{y}$	$\hat{y}$	$(y - \hat{y})$	$(y - \hat{y})^2$	$(y - \bar{y})$	$(y - \bar{y})^2$
5.20	0.90	5.20	5.03	0.17	0.03	0.00	0.00
5.00	0.90	5.20	5.03	-0.03	0.00	-0.20	0.04
5.00	1.00	5.20	5.06	-0.06	0.00	-0.20	0.04
5.20	1.10	5.20	5.09	0.11	0.01	0.00	0.00
4.90	1.20	5.20	5.13	-0.23	0.05	-0.30	0.09
5.30	1.90	5.20	5.36	-0.06·	0.00	0.10	0.01
5.50	2.10	5.20	5.42	0.08	0.01	0.30	0.09
5.50	2.30	5.20	5.49	0.01	0.00	0.30	0.09
					column sum		column sum
					(0.11)		(0.36)

- r^2 by definbition = $1 - 0.11/0.36 = 0.71$
- $(r_{y\hat{y}})^2 = 0.84^2$ (a direct computation using Excel's CORREL function) = 0.71
- $(r_{yx})^2 = 0.84^2$ (a direct computation using Excel's CORREL function) = 0.71

Fig. 5.2 Numerical illustration of r^2

denotes age. The interpretation is that mean SBP increases linearly by 1.39 as a person's age increases by 1 year. For instance, a mean SBP of 30-year-old persons is predicted as $64.30 + 1.39 \cdot 30 = 106$. This value 106 is the common systematic rule to everyone whose age = 30. Note that this regression equation should be applied for a meaningful interval of the predictor variable x (e.g., age = 200 or age = −10 is nonsense). $y = 64.30$ when $x = 0$ is indeed the y-intercept and this may not be a value of interest (i.e., for age = 0).

It is important to know that what is being predicted by this linear regression equation is the mean value of the dependent variable given a particular value of the independent variable (*aka* conditional mean). In the above blood pressure prediction example, the predicted SBP value = 106 for a given age = 30 is indeed the estimated mean SBP of all subjects with age = 30. In Fig. 5.3, the estimated regression

Fig. 5.3 Illustration of
regression mean

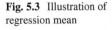

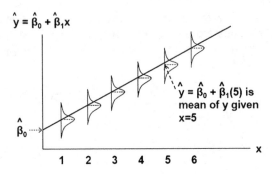

line represents the collection of predicted means (i.e., conditional means) of the dependent variable y given particular values of independent variable x.

All values on the predicted regression line are the means over the range of the given independent variable values, and a single point on that line is the estimated mean value given a particular value of the independent variable.

Many computer software programs offer to find the best (*unbiased minimum variance estimates*) regression coefficients of the specified model. Such programs also provide the estimated standard errors (SE) of the estimated regression coefficients for drawing inference. The hypothesis tests and interval estimations for the regression coefficients can be either directly available or easily completed by utilizing the computer-generated estimates.

The hypothesis test for the slope, β_1, is usually performed by a z- or t-test depending on the sample size. The practical choice of z-test is when the sample size is large enough (e.g., 30 or greater), otherwise a t-test is usually applied. The null hypothesis usually states that the regression slope is 0, i.e., H_0: $\beta_1 = 0$ (i.e., independent variable is not predictive of the outcome). The alternative hypothesis can either be nondirectional or directional depending on the research question, i.e., H_1: $\beta_1 \neq 0$ for a nondirectional test and H_1: $\beta_1 > 0$ for a directional test to claim a positive slope, etc. For both the z- and t-tests the test statistic is derived by the aforementioned "triplet," i.e., $\left[\hat{\beta}_1 - 0\right] / SE\left(\hat{\beta}_1\right)$ (see Sect. 2.2.4.5). The degrees of freedom for a t-test is $n - 2$.

The interval estimation for each regression coefficient, i.e., the slope, can be constructed using z- or t-distribution depending on the sample size. For example, the 95 % confidence interval for the regression slope β_1 with a sample size of 20 is derived as $\left[\hat{\beta}_1 - 2.101 \times SE\left(\hat{\beta}_1\right), \hat{\beta}_1 + 2.101 \times SE\left(\hat{\beta}_1\right)\right]$, where 2.101 is the t-value, of which the tail area below -2.101 is 0.025 (i.e., 2.5th percentile) and the area above 2.101 is 0.025 (i.e., 97.5th percentile) with $df = 18$. The 95 % confidence interval using z-distribution when the sample size is large enough is derived as $\left[\hat{\beta}_1 - 1.96 \times SE\left(\hat{\beta}_1\right), \hat{\beta}_1 + 1.96 \times SE\left(\hat{\beta}_1\right)\right]$.

The confidence interval (band) for the entire regression mean response line (i.e., whole collection of individual regression means given the individual values of independent variable) can also be constructed. The algebraic expression becomes more complex than that of the slope because the interval estimation for the

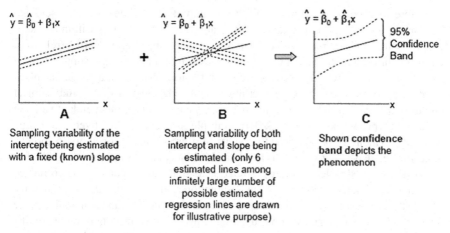

Fig. 5.4 Illustration for aiding to understand confidence interval of the estimated linear regression equation

regression line involves issues of the underlying correlation between the intercept and slope estimates that are not independent with each other. The technical details may be beyond the level of knowledge of most of the readers. Letting alone the details, Fig. 5.4 demonstrates how the confidence band appears in that the band-width around the mean of independent variable is the narrowest and becomes wider as the values of the independent variable departs from its mean. Figure 5.4a demonstrates a special situation that only the intercept is estimated while the slope is not being estimated (assumed to be known and fixed during the estimation). Intuitively, the confidence band is parallel to the estimated regression line because the slope is always fixed to one value. Figure 5.4b demonstrates the variability of estimated regression line of which both the intercept and slope are being estimated (the shown lines are only several of infinitely large number of regression lines that are estimated and fluctuating due to the sampling variability of the raw data). Then, Fig. 5.4c illustrates the actual band of a regression line. Actual calculation of this is usually done by computer software.

Another interval estimation problem is to construct a confidence interval for predicted individual outcomes. When the regression equation is applied, the point estimate of an individual outcome value at a particular value of independent variable is indeed the estimated regression mean itself which is determined at that particular value of the independent variable. However, the confidence band of the predicted individual outcome values turn out to be a little bit wider than that of the regression line (i.e., the regression mean response line) because for a point on the regression line there are many individual values surrounded randomly above and below that single mean value on a particular point of the regression line. Such a band is called prediction band (e.g., 95 % prediction band), and its computational details take into account the additional random variability of these surrounded individual observations. Actual calculation of this is usually done by computer software.

Before we proceed to the next topic, a very important issue needs to be discussed. In many applications the data are observed at multiple time points within one subject and the observations are correlated within a subject (i.e., autocorrelation). Clinical studies may include a long-time series data of only a single subject (e.g., a long-time series of weekly incidence of an infectious disease in a particular place over many years, where the particular place can be viewed as a single study subject and the dependent variable is the number of new cases and the independent variable is the number of weeks since week 0) or multiple subjects with relatively short-time series data (monthly height growth pattern of a group infants over first 6 months after life, i.e., dependent variable is height and the independent variable is month after birth). The method of least squares estimation assumes that all data are uncorrelated (i.e., there is no autocorrelation). If this assumption is violated then the standard error of the regression coefficient estimate becomes inaccurate. Advanced techniques are available, but this material will not discuss. However, it is important to ensure that whether or not the study design (or data collection mechanism) would have induced such a problem and seek statistician's guidance to resolve the problem.

5.4 Linear Regression Models with Multiple Independent Variables

The outcome (dependent) variable of a regression models may need to be explained by more than one explanatory (independent) variable. For example, gray-haired people may show higher blood pressure than the rest, but the association between age and blood pressure is probably confounded with gray hair and age association and such a phenomenon needs to be taken into account. If multiple independent variables are additionally entered into the model, the model will decrease the residual variation of dependent variable that had not been explained solely by the primary independent variable of interest. Such a model with multiple independent variables is expressed as the following linear combination (i.e., a particular value of the dependent variable given a set of values of all independent variables in the model is expressed as a weighted sum of the independent variables where the regression coefficients β's being the weights).

$$y_i = \beta_0 + \beta_1 x_1 + \beta_2 x_2 + \beta_3 x_3 + \ldots + \beta_k x_k + \varepsilon_i,$$

where the assumption about ε_i is the same as what is specified in Sect. 5.2. The predicted value of the estimated regression equation for the ith individual, i.e., $\hat{y}_i = \hat{\beta}_0 + \hat{\beta}_1 x_{1i} + \hat{\beta}_2 x_{2i} + \hat{\beta}_3 x_{3i} + \ldots + \hat{\beta}_k x_{ki}$, is the mean value of dependent variable y given the observed values of $x_{1i}, x_{2i}, x_{3i}, \ldots,$ and x_{ki}. The model fitting usually requires computer software. Below is a brief overview of how to perform such an analysis for model fitting (i.e., estimation of regression coefficients) and related inference.

The goodness of fit for a linear regression with multiple independent variables is measures by R^2 that is interpreted as the proportion of the explained variation of the

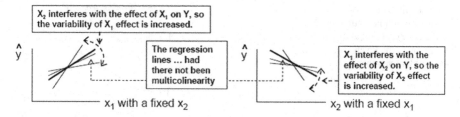

Fig. 5.5 Illustration of multi-colinearity in a multiple regression with two independent variables

dependent variable by the estimated regression equation. The least squares estimation seeks the regression coefficients that maximize and the least squares estimation seeks the regression coefficient estimates that maximize R^2. This R^2 is the squared value of the correlation coefficient between y and $\hat{y}$. In order to distinguish it from the case of simple linear regression's case (i.e., r^2), the notation uses capitalized R.

Multi-colinearity is a phenomenon due to a set of correlated independent variables in a multiple regression setting. It affects the estimated regression equation adversely. For an estimated multiple regression, $\hat{y} = \hat{\beta}_0 + \hat{\beta}_1 x_1 + \hat{\beta}_2 x_2 + \hat{\beta}_3 x_3 + \ldots \hat{\beta}_k x_k$, if two independent variables (for instance x_1 and x_2) are highly correlated, then the uncertainty about $\hat{\beta}_1$ and $\hat{\beta}_2$ increases and the standard errors of these two estimated regression coefficients are inflated. A high overall R^2 value (i.e., the independent variables, as a whole set, predict the mean outcomes pretty well) but the test results for some individual coefficients may not be significant (due to the inflated standard error of the regression coefficient estimate) and the interpretation of such regression coefficients in conjunction with other regression coefficient(s) becomes dubious (Fig. 5.5).

Exclusion of the independent variables that are highly correlated (i.e., redundant to certain variables) will prevent such an adverse consequence. A formal diagnosis can be made by using Tolerance, which is the proportion of unexplained variance of the independent variable being diagnosed by all other remaining independent variables (i.e., 1- R^2 of the estimated regression of the independent variable being diagnosed on all other variables). The inverse of Tolerance is called Variance Inflation Factor (VIF). A common criterion is to exclude the independent variable if the tolerance is less than 0.1 (or VIF greater than 10).

5.5 Logistic Regression Model with One Independent Variable: Simple Logistic Regression Model

Modeling a binary outcome variable by a regression is different from that of continuous outcome that was introduced in the previous sections. Let's discuss the following example.

Figure 5.6 illustrates a set of raw data of a set of binary outcome y (e.g., certain disease; illness if $y = 1$ and $y = 0$ if illness free) versus a continuous measure of x

Fig. 5.6 illustration of
inappropriate linear function
to predict event probability of
binary outcome given
independent variable X

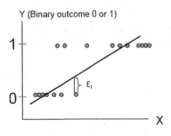

Fig. 5.7 Illustration of
logistic function to predict
event probability of binary
outcome given independent
variable X

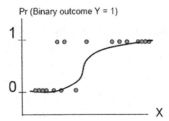

(e.g., x = age in years) in the same way that was adopted to demonstrate the single independent variable linear regression model. The linear regression line stretches out above 1 and below 0, which is unrealistic. So, the idea of forcing the feasible range lies between 0 and 1, the logistic function is adopted and Fig. 5.7 illustrates this idea.

It is noted that the observations take values of either 0 or 1 but the regression curve does not exceed either 0 or 1, and it is also noted that the vertical axis is the probability of observing $y = 1$ given a particular value of x. This is called logistic regression model because the shape of the response curve is characterized by the cumulative distribution function of the logistic distribution (simply called logistic function). The mathematical expression of this function, where **e** is the base of natural logarithm, is

$$\text{Probability } \{y = 1 \text{ given } x\} = \frac{e^{\beta_0 + \beta_1 x}}{1 + e^{\beta_0 + \beta_1 x}},$$

$$\text{and Probability } \{y = 0 \text{ given } x\} = 1 - \frac{e^{\beta_0 + \beta_1 x}}{1 + e^{\beta_0 + \beta_1 x}},$$

Unlike the linear regression model, the logistic regression model does not need the random error term because the transformed outcome variable of this logistic regression model specifies the probability of the event ($y = 1$) and this completely characterizes the probability distribution of the original outcomes of $y = 1$ and $y = 0$ (i.e., no other random error terns are necessary). A special emphasis is made here to the regression coefficient associated with the independent variable which measures the direction (positive or negative) and strength of association. Let's consider an example of which the outcome variable y is binary (1 = had an event, 0 = did not have an event) and independent variable x is a risk scale (1 = low risk, 2 = moderate risk, and 3 = high risk), the following probabilities of interests can be expressed via logistic equations:

Probability ($y = 1$ for moderate risk) = $[exp\ (\beta_0 + \beta_1 \cdot 2)]/[1 + exp\ (\beta_0 + \beta_1 \cdot 2)]$,
Probability ($y = 0$ for moderate risk) = $1 - [exp\ (\beta_0 + \beta_1 \cdot 2)]/[1 + exp\ (\beta_0 + \beta_1 \cdot 2)]$,
Probability ($y = 1$ for high risk) = $[exp\ (\beta_0 + \beta_1 \cdot 3)]/[1 + exp\ (\beta_0 + \beta_1 \cdot 3)]$, and
Probability ($y = 0$ for high risk) = $1 - [exp\ (\beta_0 + \beta_1 \cdot 3)]/[1 + exp\ (\beta_0 + \beta_1 \cdot 3)]$.

These probabilities are less of interest than the following odds ratio (OR see Sect. 1.4.3) in applied setting. If we are interested in the odds ratio of the event with high risk versus moderate risk then this odds ratio can be derived by a simple algebra as below.

$$OR = \frac{\left[Probability\left(y = 1\, for\, high\, risk\right) / Probability\left(y = 0\, for\, high\, risk\right)\right]}{\left[Probability\left(y = 1\, for\, moderate\, risk\right) / Probability\left(y = 0\, for\, moderate\, risk\right)\right]}$$

$$= \frac{\left[exp(\beta_0 + \beta_1 \cdot 3)\right]/\left[1 + exp(\beta_0 + \beta_1 \cdot 3)\right] / \left\{1 - \left[exp(\beta_0 + \beta_1 \cdot 3)\right]/\left[1 + exp(\beta_0 + \beta_1 \cdot 3)\right]\right\}}{\left[exp(\beta_0 + \beta_1 \cdot 2)\right]/\left[1 + exp(\beta_0 + \beta_1 \cdot 2)\right] / \left\{1 - exp(\beta_0 + \beta_1 \cdot 2)/\left[1 + exp(\beta_0 + \beta_1 \cdot 2)\right]\right\}}.$$

$$= exp(\beta_1 \cdot 3) - exp(\beta_1 \cdot 2) = exp(\beta_1).$$

Likewise, the OR of moderate- versus low risk is $exp\ (\beta_1 \cdot 2) - exp\ (\beta_1 \cdot 1)$, and the OR of high- versus low risk is $exp\ (\beta_1 \cdot 3) - exp\ (\beta_1 \cdot 1) = exp(\beta_1 \cdot 2) = 2 \cdot exp\ (\beta_1)$.

While the OR is the measure of association of our ultimate interest, its inference is made on the regression coefficient, β_1, because the OR is merely the transformed value of the regression coefficient (i.e., OR $= e^{\beta_1}$). The standard method for estimating the regression coefficients (i.e., fitting the logistic regression function) is the maximum likelihood (ML) method. This is a calculus approach to find the solution for the following likelihood function which is constructed by β_0 and β_1 and the observed data. The likelihood function, denoted by L, will be proportional to the joint probability of all observed events, i.e., the product of all probabilities of $y = 1$ given x for all observations with the outcome value 1 and all probabilities of $y = 0$ given x for all observations with the outcome value 0. The following is the spelled out expression of the illustrative observation set listed below.

Observation No.	Outcome y (0 or 1)	Predictor x (0 or 1)
1	1	1
2	1	0
3	1	1
.	.	.
.	.	.
.	.	.
.	.	.
n-1	0	1
n	0	0

$$L \approx \left(\frac{e^{\beta_0 + \beta_1 (x=1)}}{1 + e^{\beta_0 + \beta_1 (x=1)}} \right) \times \left(\frac{e^{\beta_0 + \beta_1 (x=0)}}{1 + e^{\beta_0 + \beta_1 (x=0)}} \right) \times \cdots \times \left(1 - \frac{e^{\beta_0 + \beta_1 (x=1)}}{1 + e^{\beta_0 + \beta_1 (x=1)}} \right) \left(1 - \frac{e^{\beta_0 + \beta_1 (x=0)}}{1 + e^{\beta_0 + \beta_1 (x=0)}} \right)$$

↑	↑	...	↑	↑
*Observation*1	*Observation*2	...	*Observationn* −1	*Observationn*
$y = 1, x = 1$	$y = 1, x = 0$		$y = 0, x = 1$	$y = 0, x = 0$

Each term in the above product is the logistic model-based probability of either $y=1$ or 0 given x. The maximum likelihood estimation procedure is a calculus problem to find the solutions for β_0 and β_1 that maximize this function. The actual computation uses its natural logarithm, $ln(L)$, instead of L by which the computation becomes much less burdensome. Letting alone the further detail of mathematical statistics aspect not addressed here, it is important and practically useful to note the property of the regression coefficients that are obtained from the ML method (*aka*, ML estimators). The property is that the sampling distribution of such an estimator follows Gaussian (i.e., normal) distribution as long as the sample size is sufficiently large. Relying on this property, similar to the simple linear regression case (see Sect. 5.2), a one-sample z-test (*aka* Wald's z-test) or t-test, if sample size is not large, is a common method for a regression coefficient β_1 to be tested for H_0: $\beta_1 = 0$ versus H_1: $\beta_1 \neq 0$. For interval estimation, the lower and upper limits of 95 % confidence interval for the regression coefficient (see Sect. 5.2) are obtained first, then these limits are transformed to OR limits, i.e., the limits are $e^{Lower\ limit\ of\ the\ regression\ coefficient}$ and $e^{Upper\ limit\ of\ the\ regression\ coefficient}$.

Because the maximum likelihood method does not resort to the least squares method, there is no goodness of fit such as the r^2 (for one independent variable) or R^2 (for multiple independent variables). Goodness of fit for an estimated logistic regression equation can be examined by several options. The most common option is to use Hosmer–Lameshow statistic, which measures the disagreement between observed versus expected events of interest in partitioned deciles (or three to nine if fewer than ten observed patterns of the independent variable(s) existed) of the predicted probabilities, and transform it to a Chi-square statistic with g-2 degrees of freedom where g is number of ordered partitions of the predicted probabilities (see Sect. 6.1).

5.6 Consolidation of Regression Models

5.6.1 General and Generalized Linear Models

Linear regression models that have more than one independent variable are called general linear models. If the regression models with more than one independent variable with its model equation is not linear (e.g., logistic) but is transformed into a linear form, then such transformed models are called generalized linear models. The meaning of "linear" is that the predicted mean value given the independent variables is expressed as a linear combination of the regression coefficients (i.e., simple addition of more than one term of which each individual term is the product of a regression coefficient and the corresponding independent variable) (see Sect. 5.2). For example, $a + bx$ is a linear combination of the two terms a and bx, and $c + dx^2$ is also a linear combination of c and dx^2. In the case of $c + dx^2$ the linearity is held between c and d. What is often confusing is that the resulting value of $c + dx^2$ turns out as a quadratic function with respect to x. However, by definition, such a regression equation is a linear model rather than a nonlinear model because the linearity between c and d is held as long as the observed x^2 value is viewed as the weight of the linear combination.

Unlike the linear models, nonlinear models are the ones that the model equation cannot be expressed by linear sum of the products created by the regression coefficients and their corresponding independent variables. For example, the logistic regression equation is a nonlinear function called logistic function (see Sect. 5.5). Nevertheless, the nonlinear function often can be converted to a linear function via algebra (i.e., linearization), and such transformed models are called generalized linear models. In the case of logistic regression, the logistic function to predict the probability of event can be transformed into a linear function to predict the log of the odds.

For the logistic regression equation Probability $\{y = 1$ given $x\} = \dfrac{e^{\beta_0 + \beta_1 x}}{1 + e^{\beta_0 + \beta_1 x}}$,

By letting *logit [p]* denote the transformation log_e [odds] $= log_e$ [$p/(1-p)$] $= log_e$ [Probability of $y=1$ given x / (1- Probability of $y=1$ given x)], the resulting equation becomes *Logit [p]* $= \beta_0 + \beta_1 x$, which is now a linear function to predict the *logit* (i.e., natural logarithm of the odds) while preserving the interpretation of both β_0 and β_1, the same as that were made in the original form, i.e., OR ($x=1$ versus 0) $= e^{\beta_1}$. Such a linearization makes the computation of the estimation less burdensome. The computational detail is beyond the objective of this monograph and is not described.

5.6.2   Multivariate Analyses and Multivariate Model

The terminologies *Multivariate Analyses* and *Multivariate Model* are very often misused by the applied researchers, and such errors appear frequently even in published articles.

A *Multivariate Analysis* is the simultaneous analysis of two or more related numeric outcome variables (i.e., dependent variables). Such methods are commonly applied in the social science research, and some popular methods are T^2-test for simultaneous comparison of two or more related means between two groups (e.g., comparison of mean weight and mean height between men and women), Multivariate Analysis of Variance (MANOVA) for simultaneous comparison of two or more related means among three or more groups (e.g., comparison of mean weight and mean height among three ethnic groups), Multivariate Regression Analysis to fit more than one correlated dependent variables by means of more than one related regression equations, Factor Analysis and Principal Component analysis to reduce a large dimension of linearly correlated variables into a small dimension, Canonical Correlation Analysis to examine a set of correlated variables with another set of correlated variables, and Linear Discriminant Analysis to build a linear equation by a set of linearly correlated random variables to differentiate the individuals into two or more groups, etc.

A *Multivariate Model* refers exclusively to a regression model of a single outcome variable with two or more independent variables (e.g., multiple linear regression models, ANCOVA models, etc.), and the analysis method is univariate because there is only one dependent variable. Note that the multiplicity of the independent variables in a model does not mean that the method is multivariate.

5.7 Application of Linear Models with Multiple Independent Variables

Figures 5.8 and 5.9 demonstrate a particular type of applications of general linear models to predict the mean of dependent variable using multiple independent variables. In the first case, the predicted mean given independent variables

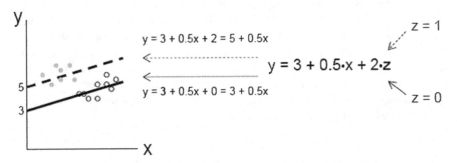

Fig. 5.8 illustration of dummy variable technique without modeling an effect of interaction

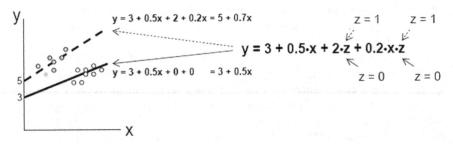

Fig. 5.9 Illustration of dummy variable technique applied to model a main effect and an effect of interaction

(i.e., regression equation) is determined by two independent variables, of which the first is a continuous variable x and the second, z, is to take either 1 or 0. Such a dichotomized independent variable to take either 0 or 1 is called dummy variable.

In Fig. 5.8 the dummy variable was used to fit the two regression lines with the same slopes but different intercepts.

In Fig. 5.9, the dummy variable was used to fit the two regression lines with two different slopes and intercepts. The last term of the regression equation is $0.2 \cdot x \cdot z$, of which the variable that takes data values is the product of x and z. Such a term is called interaction term. The corresponding regression coefficient is the size of the difference in slopes between the two subgroups of having $z = 1$ and having $z = 0$. Note that the product term variable, $x \cdot z$, is considered as a single variable (e.g., it can be renamed as any one letter variable name such as "w," etc.).

5.8 Worked Examples of General and Generalized Linear Modes

5.8.1 Worked Example of a General Linear Model

Four hundred ($n = 400$) over-weighted adults with age between 35 and 45 years participated in a 1:1 randomized 1-year study of a weight loss intervention program (i.e., 200 on the invention arm and 200 on control arm). The study collected the baseline weight and the weight change after the completion of the study.

The baseline mean (± standard deviation) weight (in lb) among all participants was 201.6 (±32.9) and their mean values of the 1-year weight changes were −3.74 (±9.34) and 4.82 (±7.12) in the intervention and control group, respectively. A general linear model analysis was applied to determine the intervention effects on the mean weight change without and with adjusting for the individual participant's age (Table 5.2 and Fig. 5.10). The dependent variable was the 1-year weight change (WC: post 1 year weight − baseline weight), and the independent variables were intervention (I: 1 = yes, 0 = no) and age (AGE: continuous. Note that intervention (I) is a dummy variable.

Table 5.2 Summary of general linear model analysis: weight loss intervention study

Model	Independent variables	$\hat{\beta}$	SE ($\hat{\beta}$)	p-Value
Model 1	Intercept	4.82	0.59	<0.0001
	Intervention (I)	− 8.56	0.83	<0.0001
Model 2, $R^2 = 0.76$	Intercept	−78.55	4.77	<0.0001
	Intervention (I)	−49.32	6.92	<0.0001
	Age (AGE)	2.09	0.12	<0.0001
	Interaction of intervention and age (I × AGE)	0.98	0.17	<0.0001

Fig. 5.10 Illustration of
effect of interaction between
intervention and age

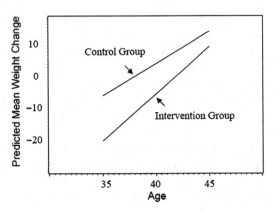

In Model 1, the estimated intercept value of 4.82 lb is the mean weight change among the control participants, and the estimated parameter value of the intervention variable (I), -8.56 ($p<0.0001$), directly offers the significant estimated difference (i.e., effect) in the mean weight changes between the two groups. With these two regression coefficients, the mean change in the intervention group can be estimated by $4.82 - 8.56 = -3.74$, which is the same as the group-specific descriptive summary statistics presented above (before performing the general linear model analysis). Model 2 was constructed in order to predict the mean weight change not only by the given intervention status but also by the age. The main effect of age as well as its interaction with the intervention (i.e., whether or not the age effects were different between the intervention and control subjects) were added to this model. Note that the estimated parameter value of the intervention (I) does not directly offer the difference in the mean weight changes between the intervention and control groups because the additional variables are included now and those effects must be taken into account simultaneously. The estimated parameter value of -49.32 ($p<0.0001$) is the group difference of the mean weight changes only for the persons with age 0. The age of 0 is unrealistic. So, if we chose a particular age of 40 for a meaningful interpretation, then the intervention group's mean weight change is predicted by $-78.55 - 49.32 \times 1 + 2.09 \times 40 + 0.98 \times 1 \times 40 = -5.07$, and that of the control group is $-78.55 - 49.32 \times 0 + 2.09 \times 40 + 0.98 \times 0 \times 40 = 5.05$, thus the estimated effect (i.e., the mean difference) at age 40 is $-5.07 - (-5.05) = -10.12$, which is the conditional effect of the intervention for 40-year-old participants. As shown in Fig. 5.10, the conditional effect decreased as the age increased.

5.8.2   Worked Example of a Generalized Linear Model (Logistic Model) Where All Multiple Independent Variables Are Dummy Variables

A large survey study investigated if the college students in California are less involved in binge drinking (Wechsler et al. 1997). The survey sample comprised

Table 5.3 Summary of generalized linear model analysis: California college students binge drinking study

Model	Independent variables	$\hat{\beta}$	SE ($\hat{\beta}$)	$\widehat{OR} = \exp(\hat{\beta})$	p-Value
Model 1	California	−0.66	0.053	0.52	<0.0001
Model 2	California	0.18	0.19	1.20	0.353
	Age < 24	0.81	0.05	2.24	<0.0001
	Male	0.44	0.03	1.56	<0.0001
	Never married	1.27	0.06	3.58	<0.0001
	White	1.08	0.05	2.95	<0.0001
	Non-commuter	0.68	0.04	1.97	<0.0001
	Smoker	1.54	0.04	4.38	<0.0001

1864 college students from California and 17,592 from elsewhere in the USA. The logistic regression analysis was performed as below.

Dependent variable – Binge drinking (1 vs. 0).

Independent variables – California student (1 vs. 0); Age < 24 (1 vs. 0); Male gender (1 vs. 0); Never married (1 vs. 0); White ethnicity (1 vs. 0); Non-commuter (1 vs. 0); Smoker (1 vs. 0) (Table 5.3).

Unlike the result summary of the general linear model (Table 5.2), the result summary of this generalized linear model analysis did not show the estimated parameter values of the intercepts (Table 5.3) because the intercept is the nuisance parameter for the odds ratio (see Sect. 5.5). The simple logistic regression model of binge drinking solely on the California residency indicator variable (1 = live in California, 0 = elsewhere) showed that there was significant decrease in binge drinking among the California college students ($\widehat{OR} = 0.52$, $p < 0.0001$). However, after simultaneously adjusting for other demographic variables and other risk factors (every variable was dichotomized as 1 = yes and 0 = no), this effect was no longer significant (Adjusted $\widehat{OR} = 1.20$, not significantly different from 1 at a 5 % significance level) while all the other covariates were significantly associated with the binge drinking in that students under 24 years old (Adjusted $\widehat{OR} = 2.24$, $p < 0.0001$), male students (Adjusted $\widehat{OR} = 1.56$, $p < 0.0001$), never married students (Adjusted $\widehat{OR} = 3.58$, $p < 0.0001$), students with white ethnic background (Adjusted $\widehat{OR} = 2.95$, $p < 0.0001$), non-commuter students (Adjusted $\widehat{OR} = 1.97$, $p < 0.0001$), and smoker students (Adjusted $\widehat{OR} = 4.38$, $p < 0.0001$) were involved more in binge drinking.

5.9   Study Questions

1. The estimated least square linear regression equation (simple or multiple regression) does not predict an individual's specific outcome value given the subject's value(s) of the independent variable(s)? What value does the regression equation predict?
2. What is the quantitative interpretation of the regression coefficient (i.e., the slope) of a least square linear regression equation?

3. What value does a logistic regression equation predict given an individual's value(s) of the independent variable(s)?
4. What is the quantitative interpretation of the regression coefficient of a logistic regression equation?
5. What are the definitions of the following?

   Odds ratio
   General linear model
   Generalized linear model

6. Explain why the multiple linear regression and multiple logistic regression are not multivariate analyses.

Bibliography

Breslow NE, Day NE (1980) Statistical methods in cancer research, vol 1, the analysis of case–control studies (IARC scientific publications no. 32). IARC, Lyon

Cox DR (1970) Analysis of binary data. Chapman and Hall, New York

Draper NR, Smith H (1998) Applied regression analysis, 3rd edn. Wiley, NJ

Hosmer DW, Lemeshow S, Sturdivant RX (2013) Applied logistic regression, 3rd edn. Wiley, Hoboken, NJ

Johnston J (1998) Econometric methods, 4th edn. McGraw-Hill, Boston, MA

MacCullagh P, Nelder JA (1989) Generalized linear models. Chapman & Hall, Boca Raton, FL

Pagano M, Gauvreau K (1993) Principles of biostatistics. Duxbury, Belmont, CA

Rosner B (2010) Fundamentals of biostatistics, 7th edn. Cengage Learnings, Inc. Boston, MA

Wechsler H, Fulop M, Padilla A, Lee H, Patrick K (1997) Binge drinking among college students: a comparison of California with other states. J Am Coll Health 45(6):273–277

Chapter 6
Normal Distribution Assumption-Free Nonparametric Inference

Methods for categorical data analysis and rank-based nonparametric methods for continuous data are discussed.

6.1 Comparing Two Proportions Using 2×2 Contingency Table

If a researcher needs to compare the binary outcome frequencies (e.g., disease rates) between two groups (e.g., risk group versus risk free group), then s/he will count the numbers and calculate the proportions (%) of observed outcomes of interest (i.e., 100 × [number of responses]/[number of subjects in each group]) and compare them. The first step is to tabulate the observed data in a 2×2 contingency table in which the four cells represent the observed number of subjects.

Figure 6.1 illustrates 2×2 contingency tables that provide information about the association between two categorical variables. The number in each cell is the observed number of subjects (i.e., cell frequency).

> *Example 6.1*
>
> Is there an association between mother's age and offspring's low birth weight?
>   Observed data (2×2 contingency table): 200 new-born infants are classified into one of the four categories (Fig. 6.2):

What should be pointed out first? Twenty percent (20 %, i.e., 10 out of 50) of the mothers who are ≤20 years old delivered low weight babies, whereas only 10 % (i.e., 15 out of 150) of the >20 years old mothers did so. A twofold difference in the risks is observed by the descriptive data summary.

H. Lee, *Foundations of Applied Statistical Methods*, DOI 10.1007/978-3-319-02402-8_6,   105
© Springer International Publishing Switzerland 2014

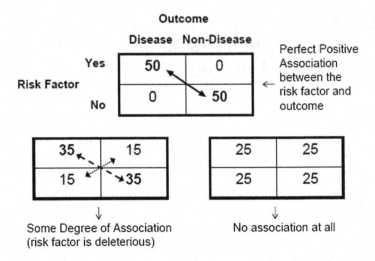

Fig. 6.1 Patterns of association between two binary outcomes

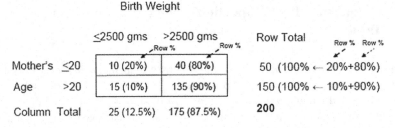

Fig. 6.2 Illustration of exploratory data analysis by contingency table

6.1.1   Chi-Square Test for Comparing Two Independent Proportions

The statistical inference to make comparison of the two independent proportions can be performed by the Chi-square test. The null and alternative hypothesis, in general, are H_0: There is no association and H_1: There is an association, respectively; or more formally,

$$H_0 : \pi_1 = \pi_2 \ \text{(There is no association between the two categorical variables)}$$

$$H_1 : \pi_1 \neq \pi_2 \ \text{(There is an association between the two categorical variables)},$$

where p_1 and p_2 denote the two population proportions. Note that the Chi-square test is always nondirectional (this will be demonstrated in the later part of this section).

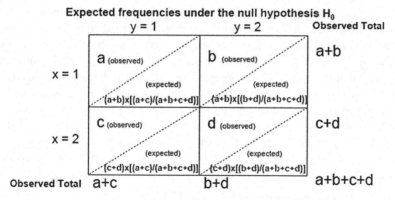

Fig. 6.3 Calculation of observed and expected counts under the null hypothesis in 2 × 2 contingency table setting

The idea is to measure discrepancy between the observed frequencies and the frequencies that are expected under the null hypothesis (i.e., there is no association) and transform the discrepancy measure to the test statistic.

As presented in Fig. 6.3, the expected frequencies of the four cells under H_0 are obtained as below. The expected frequency for the cell with $y=1$ and $x=1$ is obtained by multiplying the proportion of y=1, i.e., $(a+c)/(a+b+c+d)$, to the observed total frequency with $x=1$, i.e., $(a+b)$. Thus the expected frequency of that cell under H_0 is $(a+b) \times [(a+c)/(a+b+c+d)]$. Likewise, the expected frequencies of all four cells under H_0 are expressed as the lower entries of the cells.

Next step is to derive a test statistic that reflects the discrepancy between the observed and expected frequencies, by which we find out how likely (or unlikely) this value can happen under the null hypothesis. The value of the following expression tells you about that likelihood (or unlikelihood).

Sum of all four cell-specific values of {(Observed cell counts - Expected cell counts)²/(Expected cell counts)} will have the sampling distribution (see Sect. 2.1.2), which is close to $\chi^2_{(1)}$ distribution (Chi-square distribution with $df = 1$). This test statistic is always nonnegative because it's resulted from summing squared numbers, and it does not reflect the directionality (i.e., which observed cell frequency is more or less than the corresponding expected frequency). So, Chi-square test cannot handle directional hypotheses (i.e., always nondirectional).

In the case of Example 6.1,

Chi-square test statistic =

Sum over all four cells of {(Observed cell counts - Expected cell counts)²/(Expected cell counts)}

$= (10–6.25)2/6.25 + (40–43.75)2/43.75 +$
$(15–18.75)2/18.75 + (135–131.25)2/131.25$
$= 3.42$, and p-value = 0.06 is calculated based on $\chi^2_{(1)}$, i.e., p-value = 0.06 (Check with Excel, CHIDIST(1, 3.42) = 0.06).

Please note that in the above calculation the expected cell counts are non-integers (those were not avoidable) whereas the observed counts are obviously integers. This phenomenon lets the sampling distribution of this test statistic to only approximate (close to but not exactly the same as) $\chi^2_{(1)}$. To reduce such an approximation error, it is suggested to subtract 0.5 from the difference between each observed frequency counts and its expected frequency counts in a 2×2 contingency table (proposed by F. Yates). Such a correction prevents the researchers from overstating (i.e., reduce the chance to commit Type 1 error). In the case of Example 6.1, the continuity corrected Chi-square test statistic = *Sum over all cells of {[(Observed cell counts - Expected cell counts)-0.5] 2/(Expected cell counts)}*

$= [(10–6.25) - 0.5]2/6.25 + [(40–43.75) - 0.5]2/43.75 +$
$\quad [(15–18.75) - 0.5]2/18.75 + [(135–131.25) - 0.5]2/131.25$
$= 2.5752$ (*df*=1), *p*-value = 0.1085 by resorting to $\chi^2_{(1)}$ distribution.

Application of the continuity correction to Example 6.1 data analysis provided us a conservative result. Nonetheless, both the continuity corrected and uncorrected Chi-square statistics turned out not significant at a 5 % significance level. Thus the conclusion can be summarized as "These data showed that there was no association between mother's age and offspring's low birth weight at a 5 % significance level."

In Chap. 1, the odds ratio, OR, was introduced. The OR is also applicable in the 2×2 contingency table analysis. Note that if $\pi_1 = \pi_2$ then OR $= 1$ because $[(\pi_1/(1-\pi_1))/[\pi_2/(1-\pi_2)] = 1$, if $\pi_1 \neq \pi_2$ then OR $\neq 1$. Thus the following four pairs of null and alternative hypotheses are exchangeable.

H_0: Two proportions are equal

H_1: Two proportions are unequal

H_0: $\pi_1 = \pi_2$

H_1: $\pi_1 \neq \pi_2$

H_0: OR $= 1$

H_1: OR $\neq 1$

H_0: There is no association (between the two categorical variables y and x)

H_1: There is an association

In the case of Example 6.1, the estimated odds ratio is $[0.2/(1-0.2)]/[0.1/(1-0.1)]$ $= 2.25$, describing that the odds for an underage mother having a low birth weight baby is two-and-a-quarter times greater than that of an of-age mother. However, this was not statistically significant at a 5 % significance level.

When a directional test in a 2×2 contingency table analysis setting (e.g., H_0: π_1 $= \pi_2$ and H_1: $\pi_1 < \pi_2$) is necessary, the test can be carried out by means of a z-test. This test can be conceived as to apply independent samples z-test to compare two means where data are binary (i.e., 0 or 1). If π_1 and π_2 are not too close to 0 or 1 and the sample size is not small, this method is valid for similar reason that the probability distribution, a binominal distribution, can be approximated by the normal distribution (see Sects. 1.5.5 and 2.2.6.3).

6.1.2 Fisher's Exact Test

If there are any cells in a contingency table of which the expected frequency counts under H_0 is less than 5 (Fig. 6.4), then the sampling distribution of *Sum over all cells of {(Observed - Expected) ^{2}/(Expected)}* does not follow $\chi^2_{(1)}$ distribution, and the Chi-square test is no longer a valid test.

A special method to deal with such a situation is to directly calculate the exact probability of observing as or more extreme (i.e., departing from the null hypothesis) outcomes than the observed outcome, and then reject H_0 if the calculated exact

Fig. 6.4 Observed and expected counts in 2 × 2 contingency table

Observed Counts (Expected Counts)		Event		
		Yes	No	Total
Risk Factor	Yes	5 (2.52)	4 (6.48)	9
	No	2 (12.50)	14 (87.50)	16
	Total	7	18	25

probability is smaller than the adopted significance level (e.g., 0.05). The calculation of the exact probability (this is indeed the p-value of this exact test method) is a daunting task if carried out manually. Figure 6.5 illustrates the exact p-value calculation for the data set presented in Fig. 6.4.

Of the eight contingency tables, the third is the observed and the other seven are complete enumeration of all possible more extreme possible outcomes to both directions departing from the null hypothesis (i.e., towards deleterious and protective effects). The individual probability values that were attached to the corresponding tables are the probability of observing that particular outcomes conditional on both margins (i.e., row and column totals being fixed by the observed data). This probability is called table probability. For example, the calculation for the third table (i.e., table probability of the observed data by this study) can be spelled out as finding the chance to observe, simultaneously, 5 events out of 9 subjects with the risk factor and 2 events out of 16 subjects without the risk factor given 7 total events out of 25 study subjects, i.e., $_9C_5 \times {}_{16}C_2/_{25}C_7 = 126 \times 120/480700 = 0.0315$, where $_mC_n$ for $m \geq n > 1$ is the notation for the number of combinations of observing n events out of m, i.e., $m!/[n! \ (m-n)!]$. The remaining seven table probabilities can be calculated in the same manner.

With the calculated table probabilities of all possible enumerated tables, the p-values of the tests are calculated as below. For the directional test with its alternative hypothesis H_1: Effect is deleterious, it is intuitive (as illustrated in the Fig. 6.5) to cumulate three table probabilities that are as or more extreme to the direction of this alternative hypothesis, i.e., $0.00007489 + 0.0028 + 0.0315 = 0.0343$, indicating that there was a statistically significant deleterious effect of the risk factor at a 5 % significance level. The p-value for the other directional test, i.e., H_1: Effect is deleterious, was 0.9971, indicating that the risk factor was not protective.

For the nondirectional test, i.e., H_1: Effect is either deleterious or protective, it is also intuitive that finding the p-value is to cumulate all table probabilities that were less than or equal to that of the observed table probability in both directions, i.e., $0.00007489 + 0.0028 + 0.0315 + 0.0238 = 0.0581$.

6.1.3 Comparing Two Proportions in Paired Samples

As we apply the paired samples t-test to compare two paired means (see Sect. 3.2), when the binary outcomes are resulted from the paired samples, the application of the method introduced in Sect. 6.1.1 would no longer be valid, and McNemar's test is a valid method.

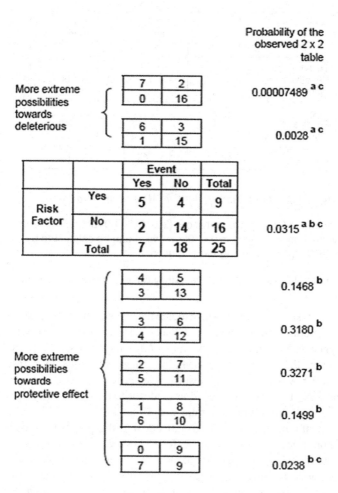

Probability of the observed 2 x 2 table

More extreme possibilities towards deleterious

7	2
0	16

0.00007489 [a][c]

6	3
1	15

0.0028 [a][c]

		Event		
		Yes	No	Total
Risk Factor	Yes	5	4	9
	No	2	14	16
	Total	7	18	25

0.0315 [a][b][c]

4	5
3	13

0.1468 [b]

3	6
4	12

0.3180 [b]

More extreme possibilities towards protective effect

2	7
5	11

0.3271 [b]

1	8
6	10

0.1499 [b]

0	9
7	9

0.0238 [b][c]

[a] Table probability to be cumulated to calculate p-value of the directional test for a deleterious effect
p-value = 0.00007489 + 0.0028 + 0.0315 = 0.0343 (i.e., sum all table probabilities that are as or more extreme than the observed towards deleterious effect)

[b] Table probability to be cumulated to calculate p-value of the directional test for a protective effect
p-value = 0.0315 + .1468 + 0.3180 + 0.3271 + 0.1499 + 0.0238 = 0.9971 (i.e., sum all table probabilities that are as or more extreme than the observed towards protective effect)

[c] Table probability to be cumulated to calculate p-value of the non-directional test for either a deleterious or a protective effect (sum all table probabilities that are less than or equal to that of the observed table)
p-value = 0.00007489 + 0.0028 + 0.0315 + 0.0238 = 0.0581

Fig. 6.5 Illustration of obtaining p-values of Fisher's exact test

	Test-2 Negative Pairs	Test-2 Positive Pairs	Total Pairs
Test-1 Negative Pairs	$n_{00} = 30$	$n_{01} = 30$	60
Test-1 Positive Pairs	$n_{10} = 10$	$n_{11} = 30$	40
Total	40	60	100

H_0: $n_{01} / (n_{00} + n_{01} + n_{10} + n_{11}) = n_{10} / (n_{00} + n_{01} + n_{10} + n_{11})$

McNemar's Chi-square statistic = $(30-10)^2 / (30+30) = 6.67$, thus p-value based on $X^2_{(1)}$ is 0.009805 which can be calculated by PROBCHI(6.67, 1) using Excel function.

Fig. 6.6 McNemar's chi-square statistic for comparing two proportions in paired samples

Let us discuss a study situation to investigate the agreement between two antibody status testing laboratory techniques, Test-1 and Test-2, which will result in either positive or negative. The summary table in Fig. 6.5 is the result of 100 pairs. Let n_{00}, n_{10}, n_{01}, n_{11} denote the number of pairs with both negative results, only Test-1 positive, only Test-2 positive, and both positive results, respectively. The ratio n_{01}/n_{10} (if $n_{01} \geq 1$ and $n_{10} \geq 1$) will depart from 1 as evidence to the discrepancy between the two test. These data showed that the ratio was 3 (i.e., $n_{01}/n_{10} = 30/10 = 3$) meaning that the discrepant outcome of Test-1 negative and Test-2 positive results occurred three times more frequently than those of Test-1 positive and Test-2 negative. Note that the number of concordant pairs is not involved in this calculation.

Let us deal with the hypothesis testing. The null hypothesis that the two tests perform the same can be written as H_0: population proportion $n_{01}/(n_{00 +} n_{01 +} n_{10 +} n_{11})$ = population proportion $n_{10}/(n_{00 +} n_{01 +} n_{10 +} n_{11})$. Under the null hypothesis, the statistic $(n_{01} - n_{10})^2/(n_{01} + n_{10})$, if $n_{01} + n_{10} > 0$, follows the Chi-square distribution with $df = 1$, $\chi^2_{(1)}$. This test is called McNemar's Chi-square Test.

These data (Fig. 6.6) showed that there was a statistically significant discrepancy between the performances of the two related test methods ($p = 0.0098$).

6.2 Normal Distribution Assumption-Free Rank-Based Methods for Comparing Distributions of Continuous Outcomes

It is true that by the Central Limit Theorem (see Sect. 2.2.2), the sample means will follow normal distributions when the sample size is large even if the sample data are drawn from a non-normally distributed population. Thus an inference

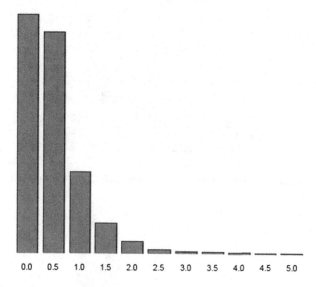

0.0   0.5   1.0   1.5   2.0   2.5   3.0   3.5   4.0   4.5   5.0

Fig. 6.7 Distribution of a population with exponential mean=0.5 and standard deviation = 0.5

about the mean using a large sample can resort to the z-test if the population standard deviation is known. Otherwise, if the population variance is unknown, then a practical choice is to substitute with the sample standard deviation and apply the t-test regardless of the sample size as we note that a t-test can be applied as long as its degree of freedom is 1 or greater (i.e., minimum sample size is 2 for a one-sample t-test for a single mean inference). Unfortunately, such an application of the t-test is valid only if it is known that the sample data were drawn from a normally distributed population. If the sample data are not drawn from a normally distributed population, then the sampling distribution of the t-statistic calculated from such data will not follow a t-distribution and the t-test is invalid. Figure 6.7 describes the distribution of a population whose distribution is not a Gaussian distribution (this is indeed an Exponential Distribution with its mean = 0.5 and standard deviation =0.5).

Figure 6.8 demonstrates the two sampling distributions of the t-statistic calculated under H_0: mean = 0.5, which are not close enough to t-distributions. The upper histogram is the result out of 100 distinct random samples, with each sample size of 5, drawn from the above population described in Fig. 6.7, and the other is that with sample size of 10. Both sampling distributions of the t-statistics calculated from small sample sizes turned out to be severely skewed to the left (i.e., not symmetric around 0 which is the expected mean of t-statistic under H_0). Note that the samples were drawn from the population with its mean = 0.5, thus the sampling distribution of those t-statistics should be symmetrical around 0 under H_0 (i.e., expected value of t under H_0 is 0).

The rest of this section will introduce alternative methods that do not require the normality assumption about the population distribution.

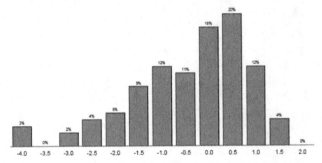

t-statistic under H_0 mean = 0.5 (sample size=5, i.e., df = 4)

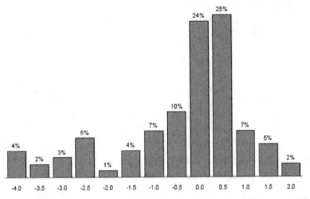

t-statistic under H_0 mean = 0.5 (sample size=10, i.e., df = 9)

Fig. 6.8 Sampling distributions of t-statistics with $n=5$ and $n=10$ based on 100 random sample data sets drawn from exponentially distributed population with mean=0.5 and standard deviation = 0.5

6.2.1   Permutation Test

The following example, using four observations in each group, demonstrates one of the normal distribution free assumption methods to examine whether or not the two independent samples are drawn from the same population.

Observed Data
Group A sample: 96, 102, 108, 126 (mean = 108)
Group B sample: 120, 128, 138, 156 (mean = 135.5)

Without knowing the probability distribution of the data, we can calculate the probability that we would observe as or more extreme (i.e., showing greater discrepancy in the two means) sample data with other permutations (see Fig. 6.9). There is only one permutation that would have made the two groups more discrepant than the observed data in the direction of Group A < Group B, and the corresponding probability is 0.029 (i.e., 2 out of 70 total permutations). This probability is indeed the p-value of the directional permutation test.

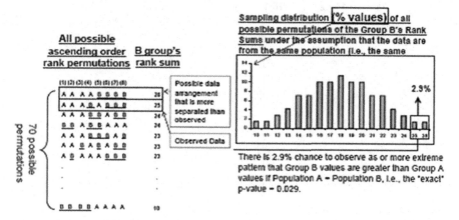

Fig. 6.9 Illustration of permutation test

6.2.2   Wilcoxon's Rank Sum Test

If data contain extreme values and the means won't be meaningful and the t-test may not perform well for comparing two independent means, what can be an alternative solution other than the permutation test of which the computational burden increases and the sample size increases? Application of t-test after data transformation (e.g., geometric mean titer analysis, etc.) can be an option, but it cannot be a universal solution. Instead, we rank the pooled (two groups are combined) data, and then apply independent samples t-test to use the rank values as the new data values. The ranking de-skews and de-extremize the extreme values so that the independent samples t-test can be applied. Such a rank-based independent samples t-test is known the same as the Wilcoxon's Rank Sum test. Wilcoxon discovered this and Mann and Whitney added mathematical work; it is also called Mann–Whitney U-test.

Figures 6.10 and 6.11 illustrate a data set for which the independent samples t-test was applied as an inappropriate method. The independent samples t-test showed that there was no significant difference in means at a 5 % significance level. Note that the observed mean difference ($Mean_1 - Mean_2$) was - 7.9, but the difference in the medians was 11.4, which may still suggest that the two sample sets were drawn from two different populations.

Figures 6.12 and 6.13 illustrate that the rank-based analysis (i.e., Wilcoxon's Rank Sum Test) would be more appropriate. The Wilcoxon's Rank Sum test showed that there was a significant difference in the two distributions at a 5 % significance level, whereas the independent samples t-test could not detect such a difference.

Group N	Mean	Median	Std Dev	Minimum	Maximum
1 25	111.3	106.7	26.1	77.2	192.8
2 25	119.2	118.1	10.9	101.3	141.9

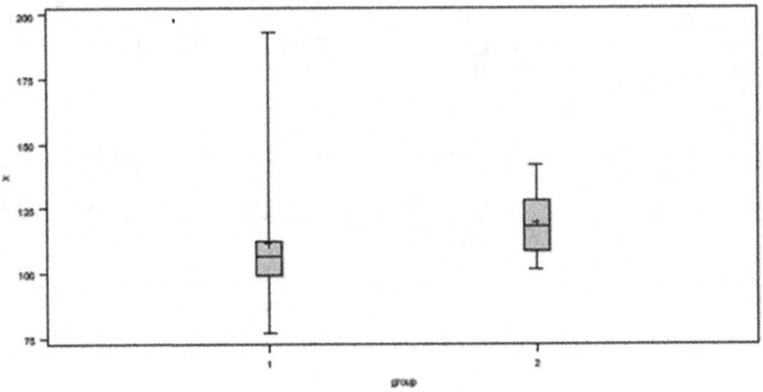

Fig. 6.10 Illustration of skewed data with unequal variations that are not suitable for an independent sample t-test

Result of Independent Samples t-test

H_o: Mean$_1$ - Mean$_2$ = 0 H_1: Mean$_1$ - Mean$_2$ is not 0

Group N	Mean	Median	Std Dev	Minimum	Maximum
1 25	111.3	106.7	26.1	77.2	192.8
2 25	119.2	118.1	10.9	101.3	141.9

Levine's Test for Equality of Variances: F (df1=24, df2=24) = 5.70, p <.0001

T-Test for	df	t-statistic	p-value
Equal variance assumption	48	-1.39	0.1708
Unequal variance assumption	32.2	-1.39	0.1739

Fig. 6.11 Illustration of data not suitable for an independent sample t-test

6.2.3   Kruskal–Wallis Test

If data are not normally distributed, the single-factor ANOVA F-test using the raw data will not work well. In such a case, we can rank the pooled data, then perform the single-factor ANOVA F-test. The rank-based single-factor ANOVA is known the same as Kruskal–Wallis Test

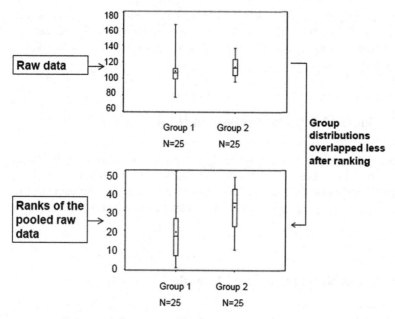

Fig. 6.12 Illustration of distributions of ranked data to apply Wilcoxon's rank sum test

Result of Wilcoxon's Rank Sum Test

Group	N	Sum of Scores	Expected Under H0	Std Dev Under H0	Mean Score
1	25	479.0	637.50	51.538820	19.160
2	25	796.0	637.50	51.538820	31.840

Wilcoxon's Rank Sum Test Statistic = 479.0, p = 0.0035

Fig. 6.13 Illustration of Wlcoxon's rank sum test

6.2.4   Wilcoxon's Signed Rank Test

If the distribution of the paired difference ($di = Bi - Ai$) is heavily skewed or contains extreme values, the mean of the paired difference won't be meaningful, and the paired samples t-test may be an inappropriate method. In such cases, we generate signed ranks of each pair-wise differences ($di = Bi - Ai$, for all i), i.e., (sign of di) × (rank of |di|), and then compute the sum of the ranks with positive sigh and that of the ranks with negative sigh, and then check discrepancy between the positively and negatively signed rank sums. A large positive (or negative) sum suggests a nonzero average difference (i.e., existence of a difference). The result of this method will be the same as that of the paired samples t-test that is applied to the generated "signed ranks." Such a signed rank-based paired samples t-test is known as Wilcoxon's Signed Rank test.

6.3   Linear Correlation Based on Ranks

We can also handle the correlation analysis between two continuous measures, say x and y, based on ranks if the data had extreme values. We assign the ranks to of x and y individual observations first, and then feed these ranks into the mathematical expression or computer program for the Pearson's Product Moment Correlation (see Sect. 5.1), *aka* Spearman's Rank Correlation.

6.4   About Nonparametric Methods

Parametric forms of inference are to estimate and test directly the parameters, and the "parameters" in this context imply the underlying probability models that generates the outcomes (i.e., beyond the constants of a particular distribution, e.g., mean and standard deviation for a Gaussian Distribution) such as Gaussian Distribution, Binomial Distribution, etc., (see Chap. 2). For continuous outcomes data, all methods of inference that were introduced in the previous chapters (e.g., t-test, ANOVA, Pearson's correlation, least square regression) require the assumption that the raw data are gathered from a Gaussian distribution (i.e., data are drawn from a normally distributed population). The word nonparametric means that the inference does not require the normality assumption. The rationale behind the nonparametric methods for continuous outcomes is to make extreme values non-extreme so that the transformed rank data appear in a "bell-like" shape, and these data can be handled by the normal distribution assumption requiring parametric methods.

What are we testing by nonparametric tests? Did this chapter mention how the null and alternative hypothesis should be articulated? Since we do not resort to the parametric distribution (i.e., the normal distribution which is completely determined by the two parameters, i.e., mean, the location parameter, and standard deviation, the dispersion parameter that tells about the spread of the distribution), the nonparametric inference does not involve an articulated hypothesis involving the parameters such as means. Now, what would be the null hypothesis of nonparametric counterpart of the independent samples t-test (i.e., Mann–Whitney's U-test or Wilcoxon's Rank Sum test)? The null hypothesis is "H_0: The two population distributions are identical," which means the two samples were drawn from the same population. The alternative hypothesis is "H_1: The two population distributions are not identical." The testing is always performed nondirectionally. Some textbooks may introduce you a null hypothesis like "the medians are the same" in that it is thought that the

Mann–Whitney's U-test or Wilcoxon's Rank Sum test compares the medians. This is mathematically true for some situations but there are many other situations where this is not exactly true depending on the particularity of the data distribution. For full apprehension of this issue, advanced knowledge of mathematical statistics is necessary, which is beyond the level and expectation of this book.

How about the Chi-square test in 2×2 contingency table setting? Does this method require data normality? No, it does not. But the probability model that generates the outcome data is a Binomial model that involves parameters (i.e., p, and n) and moreover the test statistic is Chi-square with df=1, which is a parametric distribution. Then is Chi-square a parametric or nonparametric method? Chi-square test is classified as a nonparametric method even if the data distribution is parameterized by the Binomial model and the test statistic is Chi-square with df=1. Generally speaking, "nonparametric methods" are the ones that do not require the normality of the mechanism by which the raw data were realized. More appealing name can be "raw data normality free methods."

6.5   Study Questions

1. What circumstances of the parametric inference become problematic?
2. Chi-square test for an association between two categorical variables is a non-parametric inference even if this is not a rank-based test. Why is this considered as a nonparametric inference?
3. The Chi-square test result applied to a 2×2 contingency table analysis will be consistent with that of the one independent variable logistic regression analysis by which the test for a nonzero odds ratio is performed. Why? What would be the dependent and independent variables of the logistic regression?

Bibliography

Fleiss JL (1981) Statistical methods for rates and proportions, 2nd edn. Wiley, New York
Mosteller F, Rourke REK (1973) Sturdy statistics: nonparametrics and order statistics. Addison-Wesley, Reading, MA
Pagano M, Gauvreau K (1993) Principles of biostatistics. Duxbury Press, Belmont, CA
Rosner B (2010) Fundamentals of biostatistics, 7th edn. Cengage Learnings, Inc, Boston, MA
Weerahandi S (1995) Exact statistical methods for data analysis. Springer, New York

Chapter 7
Methods for Censored Survival Time Data

7.1 Censored Observations

The following ten values are the observed survival times since diagnosis (in years) of a group of subjects with a particular cancer.

2, 4, 4+, 5, 5, 6, 6, 7+, 8+, 10

The symbol "+" indicates that the value is a censored observation meaning that the subject remained alive until that recorded time but we do not know whether or not s/he deceased thereafter. The truth is that s/he remained alive longer than the censored observation time, but there is no way to ascertain the time of death. In such a situation, what is the best way to estimate the median survival time? The next sections will guide the readers how the censored survival time data are analyzed and interpreted by the methods that take into account the censoring.

7.2 Probability of Survival Longer Than Certain Duration

Statistical descriptions and interpretations of the distribution of censored survival time are carried out by estimating the probability of survival exceeding a certain time T which is denoted by $\hat{S}(T)$. The estimate of the probability that an individual survives longer than 1 year, $\hat{S}(1)$, is obviously $\hat{S}(1) = 1$ (i.e., 100 % because all ten individuals survives longer than 1 year). The censoring did not affect this calculation. It is straightforward that the $\hat{S}(2) = 9/10$ because one subject died at time $= 2$.

Complicated calculations happen when the time of interest is 4 years or later. The idea is to calculate the probability of surviving longer than 4 years out of the individuals remaining at risk of death (i.e., have survived until then) at $T = 4$. This is conceived as the product of the two probabilities, of which the first piece is the already calculated probability of survival up to right before the time of evaluation and the second piece is the probability of survival longer than the evaluation time, i.e., $\hat{S}(4) = $ (The proportion of the subjects remaining alive longer than 2 years among all subjects) × (The proportion of the subjects remaining alive longer than 4 years among whom lived

H. Lee, *Foundations of Applied Statistical Methods*, DOI 10.1007/978-3-319-02402-8_7,   121
© Springer International Publishing Switzerland 2014

up to 4 years) = $\hat{S}(2) \times (8/9) = (9/10) \times (8/10)$. In this calculation $\hat{S}(2)$ was used as the first piece (the already calculated probability of survival up to right before the time of evaluation) because there were no deaths between 2 and 4 years. Likewise, $\hat{S}(5)$ is estimated as $\hat{S}(4) \times$ (Number of subjects remaining alive longer than 5 years among who survived after the most recent observed time of death), i.e., $\hat{S}(5) = \hat{S}(4) \times (5/7) = 0.5714$. Such a method is devised by Kaplan and Meier (Kaplan–Meier method) and is also called Product Limit method for estimating survival function. What is then the Kaplan–Meier estimate of $\hat{S}(5.5)$? Since the Kaplan–Meier survival distribution function is a step function (i.e., the values change only when the events occur), $\hat{S}(5.5)$ is still 0.5714 and it remains the same until $\hat{S}(6)$ gets updated. Applying the same idea, $\hat{S}(6) = 0.5714 \times (3/5) = 0.3428$.

The following is the completed result of Kaplan–Meier estimates:

Observed Event Times	Calculation of Kaplan-Meier Estimates	
0	$\hat{S}(0) = (10/10) = 1.0000$	1.0000
2	$\hat{S}(2) = \hat{S}(0) \times (9/10) = 0.9000$	0.9000
4	$\hat{S}(4) = \hat{S}(2) \times (8/9) = 0.8000$	0.8000
4+	$\hat{S}(4)$ remains as 0.8000 (not updated for the censored observation)	(0.8000)
5, 5	$\hat{S}(5) = \hat{S}(4) \times (5/7) = 0.5714$	0.5714
6, 6	$\hat{S}(6) = \hat{S}(5) \times (3/5) = 0.3429$	0.3429
7+	$\hat{S}(7)$ remains as 0.3429 (not updated for the censored observation)	(0.3429)
8+	$\hat{S}(8)$ remains as 0.3429 (not updated for the censored observation)	(0.3429)
10	$\hat{S}(10) = \hat{S}(6) \times (0/1) = 0.0000$	0.0000

The following is the algebraic form of the computation:

$$\hat{S}\left(\text{at } t_j\right) = \left(n_1 - d_1\right)/n_1 \times \left(n_2 - d_2\right)/n_2 \times \ldots \left(n_j - d_j\right)/n_j$$

n_j—When there is no censoring, n_i is the number of survivors just prior to time t_i. With censoring, n_i should exclude the censored cases.

d_j—d_j is the number of deaths at t_j.

Figure 7.1 describes the estimated survival distribution, which is called Kaplan–Meier Survival Curve. The graph is stepwise in that the probability of survival remains constant until the next death event is observed. The circles indicate the censored events.

7.3   Statistical Comparison of Two Survival Distributions with Censoring

The statistical inference to compare a difference between two mean survival times cannot be performed by the independent samples t-test because of the censoring even if the population survival time was normally distributed. The next example describes a very commonly used nonparametric method.

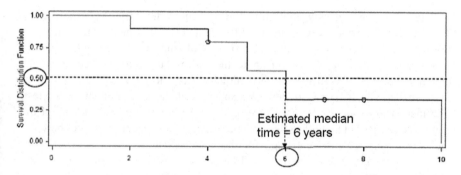

Fig. 7.1 Illustration of Kaplan–Meier survival curve and estimated median survival time

Example 7.1

Which group survived longer (survival times are recorded in years)? (Fig. 7.2)
  Group A: 2, 4, 4+, 5, 5, 6, 6, 7+, 8+, 10
  Group B: 4, 4+, 6, 6+, 6+, 9, 10, 11, 12+, 13
  Observed data summary:

Group	Total subjects	Deceased subjects	Censored subjects (%)	Median survival time (years)
A	10	7	3 (30)	6
B	10	6	4 (40)	10

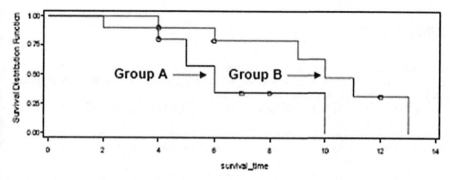

Fig. 7.2 Kaplan–Meier survival curves of two study subgroups

The inference begins with stating the null and alternative hypotheses, H_0: Two survival time distributions are not different and H_1: Two survival time distributions are different (i.e., nondirectional two-sided alternative). Note that the hypotheses did not make any statement about the means but simply stated about the distribution (i.e., the inference does not involve the location parameters of the distributions). Two statisticians, Cox and Mantel, devised a nonparametric test. The idea is to create 2×2 contingency table at every observed event time of the combined sample set that offers the evidence that the event occurrence rates between the two groups are different (e.g., for the above example, eight 2×2 tables at time$= 2$, 4, 5, 6, 9, 10, 11, and 13 will be created based on the number of each group's deceased subjects and the number of subjects remaining at risk right before the each observed event time). The test statistic cumulates the individual 2×2 table's Chi-square values calculated from those 2×2 tables under H_0. The sampling distribution of this test statistic approaches to the Chi-square distribution with $df = 1$ as the sample size becomes sufficiently large. This test was called Log-Rank Test later by two statisticians, Peto and Peto. The name *Log-Rank Test* reveals the technical aspect of how the test statistic is devised (interested readers should read Peto and Peto 1972; also see References of Chap. 7).

The result of the test obtained from a computer software was that the Log-rank Chi-square ($df = 1$) was 3.9016 with a p-value of 0.0482, which can be summarized as "These data showed that the survival times of the two populations were significantly different ($p = 0.0482$)."

7.4 Study Question

1. Explain the product limit calculation for estimating a survival time distribution. What are the individual probabilities being multiplied?

Bibliography

Cox DR, Oakes D (1984) Analysis of survival data. Chapman & Hall, London
Lee ET, Wang J (2003) Statistical methods for survival data analysis, 3rd edn. Wiley, New York
Miller RG (1981) Survival analysis. Wiley, New York
Peto R, Peto J (1972) Asymptotically efficient rank invariant test procedure. J R Stat Soc Ser A 135(2):185–207
Rosner B (2010) Fundamentals of biostatistics, 7th edn. Cengage Learnings, Boston, MA
Smith PJ (2002) Analysis of failure and survival data. Chapman & Hall, Boca Raton, FL

Chapter 8
Sample Size and Power

8.1 Sample Size for Interval Estimation of a Single Mean

For single mean interval estimation of a $100 \times (1-\alpha)\%$ confidence interval, e.g., for $\alpha = 0.05$, $100 \times (1-0.05)\% = 95\%$, the width of the interval is a function of several elements, among which the pivotal one is the sample size.

As discussed in Sect. 2.2.6.2, the following steps derive the sample size for a 95% confidence interval using Gaussian approximation (i.e., resort to the C.L.T. for approximating the sample distribution of the sample mean to a Gaussian distribution, see Sect. 2.2.2); in that the first step is to set up an equation by letting one-half of the width (an error margin of $w/2$) be equal to the distance of the 97.5th percentile from the mean of the standard normal distribution $\times$ the standard error of the sample mean, i.e., $w/2 = 1.96 \times s/\sqrt{n}$, where s denotes the sample standard deviation, then solve this equation for n. The final equation will be $n = (3.92 \times s/w)^2$. As depicted in Fig. 8.1, the interval becomes narrower as the sample size increases (i.e., inversely proportional to $\sqrt{n}$).

The following example aids to understand how the required sample size is determined for constructing a 95% confidence interval for one mean inference.

Example 8.1

Standard dosage level of medication "A" will lower the heart rate over 48 h. A new study for a higher dose is being proposed, and the investigator wants to determine how many study subjects do enroll into this study; of which resulting data would provide a 95% CI of the mean heart rate that is not wider than 5 bpm if the anticipated sample standard deviation is $s = 10$ bpm?

Given $w = 5$ and $s = 10$;

Solve $w/2 = 1.96 \times 1/\sqrt{n}$ for n;

H. Lee, *Foundations of Applied Statistical Methods*, DOI 10.1007/978-3-319-02402-8_8,   125
© Springer International Publishing Switzerland 2014

$n = (3.92 \cdot s/w)^2 = (3.92 \cdot 10/5)^2 = 61.5;$

Sample size $= 62$

If the study subject recruitment is not difficult then 62 patients can be a generously determined sample size. It is also possible to curtail the sample size to the integral part of the solution (i.e., do not need to round up to save the resource), i.e., $n = 61$ which would not have a large impact.

How many more subjects do we need if we want to shrink the length of the 95 % CI down to no more than 4 bpm?

$n = (3.92 \cdot s/w)^2 = (3.92 \cdot 10/4)^2 = 96.04$

Sample size $= 96$, thus 34 more patients are required.

Note that in order to decrease the error margin by 20 %, 34 more patients are required which is an increase of 55 %, not the same increase of 20 %.

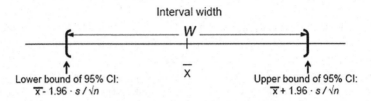

Fig. 8.1 Sample size determination for interval estimation of a single mean

8.2 Sample Size for Hypothesis Tests

8.2.1 Sample Size for Comparing Two Means Using Independent Samples z- and t-Tests

As discussed in Sect. 2.2.4, the sample size required for a hypothesis testing to compare two independent means depends on:

1. Level of significance (α)
2. Power ($1-\beta$), where β is the probability of committing type-2 error
3. Alternative hypothesis (1- or 2-sided)
4. Size of detectable difference in means (δ)
5. Standard deviation of the outcome distribution under the null hypothesis (σ)

The idea of determination of required sample size for comparing two means using independent samples z-test is illustrated in Fig. 8.2, which depicts the relationship between the sample size and the five determinants. The two density curves describe the sampling distributions of test statistic z under H_0 (left curve) and H_1 (right curve). Note that the right-hand side curve is a snap shot of the horizontally

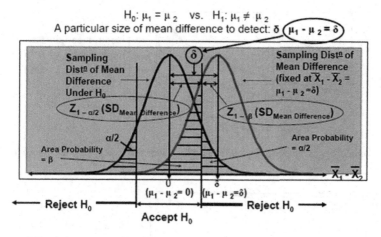

Detectable Difference in Means (δ)

$$\frac{\text{Detectable Difference in Means } (\delta)}{\sqrt{(\sigma^2/n_{group1} + \sigma^2/n_{group2})}} = Z_{1-\alpha/2} + Z_{1-\beta} \longrightarrow \text{Solve for } n_{\text{per group}}$$

Fig. 8.2 Sample size for a nondirectional hypothesis test for comparing two means using normal approximation, i.e., independent samples z-test. *Note*: $\sqrt{(\sigma^2/n_{group1} + \sigma^2/n_{group2})} = SD_{MeanDifference}$ (i.e., standard error of the mean difference) and σ^2 denotes the population variance of each group—we assume that the variances are equal (i.e., σ^2 is a common variance); $n_{group1} = n_{group2} = n_{\text{per group}}$ because we consider a balanced design

sliding curve that stopped (for illustration) where the alternative hypothesis' mean difference is a certain non-zero value δ.

Within the rejection region, the null- and alternative distributions overlapped. The shaded area under the null distribution is the size of type-1 error and the area under the alternative distribution is the power.

Left-hand side of the equation is the standardized (standard deviation unit of the sampling distribution of the mean difference) effect size. Right-hand side of the equation spells out the left-hand side into a sum of the following two parts: (1) the distance between the null mean and the critical value of the test on the z-scale and (2) the distance between the critical value and the alternative mean value of the test on the z-scale. Finally this equation is solved for the sample size per group.

$$n \text{ per group} = 2\left\{\frac{\sigma \times (z_{1-\alpha/2} + z_{1-\beta})}{\text{Detectable difference in means}, \delta}\right\}^2$$

Note that σ is the common standard deviation of the two population distributions which are assumed to have the same standard deviation, and that β is specified (instead of $\beta/2$) although this is a nondirectional test because of the fixed δ the left tail area of the alternative distribution covered by the other side of the rejection region is nearly zero, and also note that n is the sample size per group, not the study sample size.

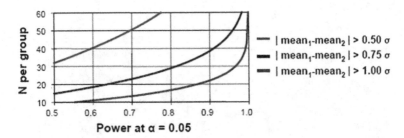

Fig. 8.3 Sample size given power and effect size for independent samples z-test for comparing two means

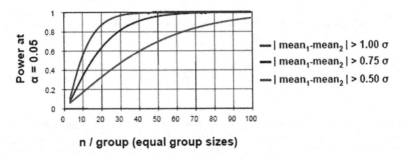

Fig. 8.4 Power given sample size and effect size for independent samples z-test for comparing two means

As illustrated in Fig. 8.3, the required sample size increases geometrically as the targeted power increases and the targeted effect size decreases.

As illustrated in Fig. 8.4, the power is proportional to the square root of the given sample size and inversely proportional to the square root of the effect size.

Example 8.2

A sample size determination is needed for a nondirectional z-test, with its power = 80 % at an adopted significance level, α, of 5 %, to compare the mean systolic blood pressures between the two independent groups, Group A and Group B. A pilot data suggested that the means are approximately 132.86 and 127.44 in Group A and Group B, respectively (i.e., difference size = 132.86 - 127.44 = 5.42) and the known common population $\sigma = 16.8$. What should be an adequate sample size to detect a mean difference of 5.42?

For a nondirectional test with its adopted significance level, $\alpha = 0.05$, power to attain, $1 - \beta = 0.8$, and the common population standard deviation, $\sigma = 16.8$, the sample size per group for a balanced design (i.e., equal group size) is determined by the aforementioned equation

$$n \text{ per group} = 2 \left\{ \frac{\sigma \times \left(z_{1-\alpha/2} + z_{1-\beta}\right)}{\text{Detectable difference in means}, \delta} \right\}^2,$$

where $z_{1-\beta} = z_{0.8} = 0.84$ (i.e., z-value of the area under the standard Gaussian density curve covering from negative infinity to 0.8, and this can be found by using the Excel function NORMSINV(0.8) = 0.84).

Similarly $z_{1-\alpha/2} = z_{1-0.025} = z_{0.975} = 1.96$ (using the Excel function NORMSINV(0.975) = 1.96), and the difference in means to detect is 5.42 (about one-third of σ). The solution of the equation is 151, i.e., n per group = 2 $\{16.8 \times (0.84 + 1.96)/5.42\}^2 = 151$.

Let us now consider the independent samples t-test to compare two means when the population standard deviation is not known under the assumption that the data are drawn from normally distributed populations. The principle of sample size determination is almost the same as that of the z-test except that the sampling distribution of the test statistic is t-distribution which is a little bit more difficult to deal with. The difficult part is that the sampling distribution of the test statistic, t, under the alternative hypothesis must be characterized by not only the two means and standard error of the mean difference but also by two more parameters. These two parameters cannot be known until the sample size is known, so, unlike the z-test case, the sample size determination cannot be achieved by solving a single closed form equation of which the sample size being sought is not the one and only unknown variable. The first of these two parameters is the degree of freedom, df. As we already learned in the previous chapters that the degree of freedom is dependent on the sample size being sought. The other is the non-centrality parameter. The non-centrality parameter corresponds to the standardized effect size of the test

$$\frac{\text{Detectable Difference in Means}(\delta)}{\sqrt{\left(\sigma_{group1}^2 / n_{group1} + \sigma_{group2}^2 / n_{group2}\right)}}.$$

In the t-test setting, the population standard deviations, σ_{group1} and σ_{group2}, are unknown but can be replaced with the sample standard deviations s_{group1} and s_{group2} for approximation. In any event, without this parameter being known, the sampling distribution of the test statistic t under the alternative hypothesis cannot be completely characterized. Obviously, the sampling distribution under the null hypothesis of equal means explicitly determines its non-centrality parameter to be zero, thus the sampling distribution of t under the null hypothesis is also called a central t-distribution. As illustrated in Fig. 8.5, unlike the z-test, the sampling distribution of the t-statistic under the alternative hypothesis has larger variation (degree of freedom of 18, i.e., sample size = 20, non-centrality parameter = 3.5, reject H_0: $\mu_1 = \mu_2$ if $t < -2.1$ or $t > 2.1$ in favor of the nondirectional alternative hypothesis H_1: $\mu_1 \neq \mu_2$) than that under the null hypothesis. Of course, the degree of increase in the variation for a fixed non-centrality parameter is also dependent on the degree of freedom (i.e., the sample size being sought). Such an interconnection makes the sample size determination more complicated than that of the z-test.

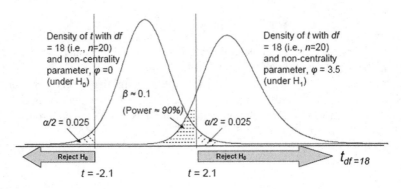

Fig. 8.5 Power of a nondirectional hypothesis test for comparing two means using independent samples t-test

For this reason, the sample size can be determined iteratively, in that a rough estimate of the sample size is fixed temporarily to calculate the resulting power based on the non-central t-distribution characterized by the alternative hypothesis and continue to update the sample size until the resulting power is close enough to the targeted power. Computer programs as well as the calculated power tables for t-tests given a wide range of predetermined sample size, non-centrality parameter (or difference in means), sample standard deviations of the two groups, and level of significance, α, are widely available.

Comment on non-centrality parameter and beyond: We had not introduced the non-centrality parameter to the t-distribution until we encounter the situation for calculating the power of a test using a specified sampling distribution of the test statistic, t, under an alternative hypothesis. This parameter does not influence the sampling distribution under the null hypothesis, and so is the practical aspect of carrying out a t-test, i.e., calculation of the p-value and/or determining the critical region as long as the directionality (one- or two sided) of the alternative hypothesis is only specified. The non-centrality parameter was necessary in the calculating the power given the significance level, α, and the known sample size. The power calculations for the Chi-square- and F-test also require the non-centrality parameters of these sampling distributions under the alternative hypotheses. Involvement of the non-centrality parameter in Chi-square- and F-distributions is due to the fact that both distributions are derived in relation with t-distribution. Interested readers may learn the mathematical genesis of Chi-square- and F-distributions and the power calculation problem for estimating a sample size given the significance level, α, the alternative hypothesis, and the known sample size from further readings such as Winer (1971).

8.2.2   Sample Size for Comparing Two Proportions

The Chi-square test is commonly used to compare two independent proportions in 2×2 contingency table analysis setting. However, because of the complexity to deal

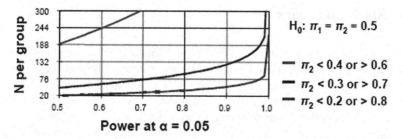

Fig. 8.6 Sample size given power and effect size for independent samples z-test for comparing two proportions

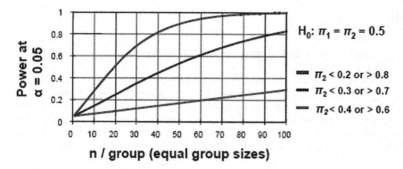

Fig. 8.7 Power given sample size and effect size for independent samples z-test for comparing two proportions

with the non-centrality discussed in § 8.2.1, and also because the sampling distribution of the square root of the Chi-square statistics under the null hypothesis for the 2×2 contingency table analysis is the same as that of the z-distribution (see § 6.1.1), the sample size can be determined by a method very similar to that of the independent samples z-test for comparing two means. The following equation determines the sample size per group in a balanced design (i.e., equal group size) which is derived based on the z-distribution (i.e., normal approximation of Binomial Distribution) (see Sect. 1.5.5) wherein π_A and π_B indicate the two independent proportions under alternative hypothesis, α is the adopted significance level, and β is the size of the power to attain.

$$n \, \text{per group} = \left\{ \frac{\left[2\pi_A\left(1-\pi_A\right)\right]^{1/2} z_{1-\sigma/2} + \left[\pi_A\left(1-\pi_A\right)\right] + \left[\pi_A\left(1-\pi_B\right)\right]^{1/2} z_{1-\beta}}{\text{Detectable difference in proportions}} \right\}^2$$

Figures 8.6 and 8.7 present the relationship among sample size, power, and effect size at an adopted 5 % significance.

8.3   Study Questions

1. Explain why the graphs of Figs. 8.3 and 8.4 do not appear as straight lines.
2. An investigator determined a sample size for a new study to detect a certain effect size (difference in two means) with 80 % power at a 5 % significance level using an independent samples t-test. If this investigator chooses a smaller effect size, then the sample size will have to increase. If a newly chosen effect size became its half size of the previously determined sample size without altering the power and significance level of the test, then should the new sample size be doubled or quadrupled?

Bibliography

Chow SC, Wang H, Shao J (2002) Sample size calculations in clinical research, 2nd edn. Chapman & Hall, Boca Raton, FL
Le CT (1992) Fundamentals of biostatistics inference. Marcel Dekker, New York
Rosner B (2010) Fundamentals of biostatistics, 7th edn. Cengage Learnings, Boston, MA
Sahai H, Khurshid A (1996) Formulae and tables for the determination of sample sizes and power in clinical trials for testing differences in proportions for the matched pair design: a review. Stat Med 15:1–21
Winer BJ (1971) Statistical principles in experimental design, 2nd edn. McGraw-Hill, New York

Chapter 9
Review Exercise Problems

9.1 Review Exercise 1

1. A measure of body temperature (°F) is _____. Which answer is correct (5 points)?

   (1) An interval datum
   (2) A ratio datum
   (3) A discrete datum
   (4) A continuous datum

   (a) None of these
   (b) Only (1)
   (c) Only (2)
   (d) Only (3)
   (e) Only (4)
   (f) (1) & (2)
   (g) (1) & (3)
   (h) (1) & (4)
   (i) (2) & (3)
   (j) (2) & (4)
   (k) (3) & (4)
   (l) (1) & (2) & (3)
   (m) (1) & (2) & (4)
   (n) (1) & (3) & (4)
   (o) (2) & (3) & (4)
   (p) (1) & (2) & (3) & (4)

2. In a normal distribution _____. Which answer is correct (5 points)?

   (1) The mean, median, and mode are the same.
   (2) The interval from half standard deviation below the mean to half standard deviation above the mean (i.e., mean - $0.5 \times$ SD ~ mean + $0.5 \times$ SD interval) covers approximately 38.3 % of the distribution.

H. Lee, *Foundations of Applied Statistical Methods*, DOI 10.1007/978-3-319-02402-8_9,   133
© Springer International Publishing Switzerland 2014

(3) The interval from 1.96 standard deviation units below the mean to 1.96 standard deviation units above the mean (i.e., mean - $1.96 \times SD \sim$ mean $+ 1.96 \times SD$ interval) covers 97.5 % of the distribution.

   (a) None of these
   (b) Only (1)
   (c) Only (2)
   (d) Only (3)
   (e) (1) & (2)
   (f) (2) & (3)
   (g) (1) & (3)
   (h) (1) & (2) & (3)

3. In the t-distribution with $df = 20$ and non-centrality parameter $= 0$, _____. Which answer is correct (5 points)?

(1) The mean, median, and mode are the same.
(2) The interval from -1.725 to 1.725 covers 95 % of t-values.
(3) The interval from -2.528 to 2.528 covers 95 % of t-values.
(4) The interval from -2.086 to 0.000 covers 47.5 % of t-values.

   (a) None of these
   (b) Only (1)
   (c) Only (2)
   (d) Only (3)
   (e) Only (4)
   (f) (1) & (2)
   (g) (1) & (3)
   (h) (1) & (4)
   (i) (2) & (3)
   (j) (2) & (4)
   (k) (3) & (4)
   (l) (1) & (2) & (3)
   (m) (1) & (2) & (4)
   (n) (1) & (3) & (4)
   (o) (2) & (3) & (4)
   (p) (1) & (2) & (3) & (4)

4. In the F-distribution (under the null hypothesis for an ANOVA F-test) with $df_{numerator} = 3$ and $df_{denominator} = 5$ _____. Which answer is correct (5 points).

(1) The mean, median, and mode are the same.
(2) The probability of observing a value of $F > 5.41$ is 0.025.
(3) The smallest possible value is 0.
(4) The square root of F (dfnumerator $= 3$, dfdenominator $= 5$) $= t$ (df $= 5$).

   (a) None of these
   (b) Only (1)
   (c) Only (2)

(d) Only (3)
(e) Only (4)
(f) (1) & (2)
(g) (1) & (3)
(h) (1) & (4)
(i) (2) & (3)
(j) (2) & (4)
(k) (3) & (4)
(l) (1) & (2) & (3)
(m) (1) & (2) & (4)
(n) (1) & (3) & (4)
(o) (2) & (3) & (4)
(p) (1) & (2) & (3) & (4)

5. The power refers to _____. Which is answer is correct (5 points)?

   (1) Probability of rejecting the null hypothesis when it is false.
   (2) 1 minus the probability of type-1 error.
   (3) The size of the difference between the values stated in the null hypothesis and the alternative hypothesis.
   (4) 1 minus p-value.

      (a) None of these
      (b) Only (1)
      (c) Only (2)
      (d) Only (3)
      (e) Only (4)
      (f) (1) & (2)
      (g) (1) & (3)
      (h) (1) & (4)
      (i) (2) & (3)
      (j) (2) & (4)
      (k) (3) & (4)
      (l) (1) & (2) & (3)
      (m) (1) & (2) & (4)
      (n) (1) & (3) & (4)
      (o) (2) & (3) & (4)
      (p) (1) & (2) & (3) & (4)

6. Please make the stem-and-leaf plot of the following 11 observations (5 points):
   41 48 51 52 55 56 58 63 65 67 83

7. Dr. Z studied 28 patients with a certain chronic illness. From the patients' history review, the means and the variances of the ages at the occurrence of first episode for the severe, moderate, and mild groups are summarized in the following table. Please note that these data are not real, but they were made up for an easy calculation.

Descriptive statistics for problems 7.1–7.16		
	Mean age	Variance of age distribution
Severe (group 1) (**n=10**)	30.00	25
Moderate (group2) (**n=10**)	35.00	25
Mild (group 3) (**n=8**)	41.25	25

7.1–7.4 Based on the past experience, Dr. Z suspected that the mean age of first episode occurrence within the severe group would be 33 or less (i.e., younger). Please perform a *t*-test at a 5 % significance level.

7.1. Stating null and alternative hypotheses

(A) Write up a proper null hypothesis that should have been written prior to the data collection (please do not use mathematical notations but do verbalize) (1 point).

(B) Write up the alternative hypothesis that negates your stated null hypothesis that should have been written prior to the data collection (please do not use mathematical notations but do verbalize) (1 point).

7.2. Test statistic

(A) Calculate the numerator of your *t*-statistic under the null hypothesis which is (observed severe group's mean age at occurrence of the first episode for the severe – the mean under the null hypothesis) (1 point).

(B) Calculate the denominator of the *t*-statistic which is the standard error of the numerator, i.e., SE of (observed severe group's mean age at occurrence of the first episode for the severe – the mean under the null hypothesis) (4 points).

(C) What is the value of your observed *t*-statistic (2 points)?

7.3. Determination of the significance
You can either calculate the *p*-value directly or determine the critical region first then determine if the observed test statistic is within the critical region of the sampling distribution under the null hypothesis. The degree of freedom of your test statistic's distribution is 9.

(A) If you decided to calculate the *p*-value using Excel, which Excel function would you use? _____ (1 point)

(B) Please determine the *critical region* of this test (note: a critical region is not simply the critical cutoff value/values of the test statistic *t*). _____ (2 points)

(C) *p*-value of the observed test statistic *t*: _____

7.4. Write a single sentence that can go into the results section of a research paper. Please *do not* write a sentence like "The null hypothesis was rejected because ....." (2 points).

7.5–7.8 Please perform a *t*-test at a 5 % significance level to examine if the mean ages of the first episode occurrence are the same in both severe patients and moderate patients or otherwise the severe patients encounter their first episode *sooner* in life than the moderate patients.

7.5. Stating null and alternative hypotheses

   (A) Write up a null hypothesis that should have been written prior to the data collection (please do not use mathematical notations but do verbalize) (1 point).

   (B) Write up the alternative hypothesis that negates the null hypothesis that should have been written prior to the data collection (please do not use mathematical notations but do verbalize) (1 point).

7.6. Test statistic

   (A) Calculate the numerator of the *t*-statistic, i.e., observed mean difference − expected mean difference under the null hypothesis. Mean difference set up: [severe group's mean − moderate group's mean] (1 point).

   (B) Calculate the denominator of the *t*-statistic which is the standard error of the numerator, i.e., SE of (observed mean difference − expected mean difference under the null hypothesis) (5 points).

   (C) If you carried out (A) and (B) correctly, then the *t*-statistic is −2.236. Please show your derivation (simply follow "*triplet*" set up found in Sect. 3.1) (4 points)?

7.7. Determination of the significance using
   You can either calculate the *p*-value directly or determine the critical region first then examine whether or not the observed test statistic is within the critical region. The degree of freedom of your test statistic's distribution is 18.

   (A) If you decided to calculate the *p*-value using Excel, which Excel function would you use? _____ (1 point).

   (B) Please determine the *critical region* of this test (note: a critical region is not simply the critical cutoff value/values of the test statistic *t*). _____ (1 point).

   (C) *p*-value: _____ (2 points).

   (D) In order for the difference becomes significant at the chosen significance level, what should be the smallest value of the difference? (4 points).

7.8. Confidence interval of the mean difference

   (A) Using a *t*-distribution, please construct a 90 % confidence interval on the difference between the two means (i.e., severe mean age − moderate mean age). Please carry out this calculation as instructed (i.e., do not calculate either moderate mean age - severe mean age or take an absolute value of the result).

   (B) Write a single sentence that can go into the results section of a clinical journal paper (2 points).

7.9–7.14 The following ANOVA table is constructed to compare the mean ages of first episode onset among the three groups (i.e., H_0: All three means are equal vs. H_1: At least one mean is different from the rest).

Please complete the table. Note that you need to calculate the grand mean age, and please be careful with that calculation.

Source	df	Sum of squares	Mean squares	F value
Between severities	2	7.9 ____(3 pts)	7.12 ____(1 pt)	7.14 ____(1 pt)
Error (within severity)	25	7.10 ____(3 pts)	7.13 ____(1 pt)	
Total	27	7.11 ____(1 pt)		

7.15. Calculate the p-value using Excel (2 points).

7.16. Write a single sentence that can go into the results section of a clinical journal paper (2 points).

7.17. Dr. Z plans on constructing a new study (Z-10 study) that will enroll only the severe and moderate patients. The plan is to enroll 200 patients in each group in order to detect a smaller difference than what was observed in the above small Z-09 study (note that Z-09 study showed a difference of 5 years in mean ages). The inference will be a directional independent samples z-test at a 5 % significance level with a 90 % power. It is known that the population variances of the three groups are known and equal to 25. Please provide a reasonable approximation of the minimum detectable statistically significant difference between the two mean ages (your answer should include the wording "a difference in mean ages of at least ____ years") for Z-10 study. Please show fully annotated work including the justification for some assumptions or subjective decision that you might have made (5 points).

8. Dr. A at a major university affiliated teaching hospital conducted a pilot efficacy study to investigate whether or not a new post-surgery rehabilitation intervention can improve patient quality of life during a 4-week period after a hip surgery (A-01 study). The study was a two-arm (conventional versus new intervention groups) randomized study. The sample size of this A-01 study was determined to detect at least $m\%$ greater improvement in the mean score among the patients receiving the new intervention at a 10 % significance level with a power of 80 % by a directional t-test. Dr. A assumed equal variance and the common standard deviation value that Dr. A used for the sample size determination was $s\%$. The study enrolled 15 patients receiving the intervention and 15 patients receiving traditional intervention (total sample size of 30). The result of A-01 study was quite promising in that the directional statistical test (i.e., independent samples t-test) was significant at the predetermined significance level of 10 % (it is not uncommon that a pilot study chooses a lenient significance level than 5 %); and the patients who received the new intervention showed that the mean percentage improvement of the physical strength subscale of SF-36 quality of life scale was greater by about $m\%$ after 4 weeks.

Based on the A-01 study, Dr. A suspected that a new study could detect even a smaller difference; and he proposed a new study (A-02 study) that will enroll 60 patients per group (i.e., total study sample size of 120). In the sample size determination section of the A-02 study proposal, Dr. A justified that the proposed sample size is adequate to show a statistically significant mean percentage improvement in the subscale by at least $m/2\%$ by using a directional independent sample t-test at a 5 % significance level with a power of 80 %. The common standard deviation of the mean percentage improvement remains the same as that of study A-01.

Question: Was Dr. A's sample size justification reasonable? Why/why not? (5 points)

9. Which of the following is true? (5 points).

(1) The distribution of a random sample data set drawn from a non-normal continuous population distribution will approach to a normal distribution as the sample size becomes very large.
(2) The distribution of sample means obtained from a non-normal continuous population distribution will approach to a normal distribution as the sample size becomes very large.
(3) The distribution of the sample means obtained from a normal population distribution will approach to a normal distribution as the sample size becomes very large.

   (a) None of these
   (b) Only (1)
   (c) Only (2)
   (d) Only (3)
   (e) (1) & (2)
   (f) (2) & (3)
   (g) (1) & (3)
   (h) (1) & (2) & (3)

9.2   Review Exercise 2

9.2.1   Part A (30 Points): Questions 1–15 "True/False" Questions, Please Explain/Criticize Why If You Chose to Answer False (2 Points Each)

1. Coefficient of variation (CV) can measure the variability of data measured on the interval or ratio scale and is useful to compare the variations of two different characteristics of the same patient group measures in the same unit or those of the same characteristics from two or more different patient groups. (True/False).

2. A large size statistics course class' final test scores are normally distributed. CV of the test score distribution is 10 % and the average score is 80. It can be interpreted that approximately 31.7 % of the students received their scores either above 88 or below 72 (i.e., outside of these two high and low scores). (True/False).

3. Mean (± standard deviation) of pulse rate of a large group of people is known as 65 beats/min (±10). It is also known that the pulse rate of this group is normally distributed. The proportion of the people with pulse rate over 85 beats/min is approximately less than 5 % but greater than 2 % (i.e., 2 %<pulse rate<5 %). (True/False).

4. A researcher conducted a small study (n = 15) and estimated a sample mean and its standard error of a continuous measurement, then constructed a normal approximation based 95 % confidence interval around the population mean. The result was presented to a department's seminar. Another researcher made a comment that the confidence interval would be slightly wider if it had been constructed based on the t-distribution with $df = 14$. (True/False).

5. Dr. Z proposed a comparative study involving a total of 60 study subjects of whom 30 subjects will receive medication A and the other 30 will receive placebo. He wants to detect a 10-point reduction in mean pain scale score among the subjects on medication A compared to the mean of the placebo subjects by using the directional independent samples t-test at a 5 % significance level with 80 % power. A reviewer agreed with the choice of the t-test. However, it is criticized that the detectable difference is too large and a 5-point reduction is needed to be detected. Then the researcher decided to double the study sample size (i.e., a total of 120 subjects) to detect at least 5 points reduction in mean pain score by the same test (i.e., directional independent samples t-test, the same power, the same significance level, and the same assumption about the standard deviation). Dr. Z's decision was correct. (True/False).

6. If a hypothesis test did not show a statistically significant difference in two means but the observed difference in the two sample means was large enough, we should not exclude a possibility that the study had been underpowered. (True/False).

7. An investigator wants to perform a hypothesis test of which H_0: Mean = 100 and H_1: Mean > 100. It is observed that the sample mean = 100 and its standard error = 50 from a random sample set of size 10 drawn from a normally distributed population. A t-test is not applicable because the t-test is only applicable in a two-group comparison or a paired mean comparison. (True/False).

8. If a t-distribution based 95 % confidence interval on a difference in two means excluded 0 and the signs of the upper and lower confidence limits were the same and they were in the desirable direction, we can say that the nondirectional independent samples t-test for the comparison would also reject H_0: $mean_1 = mean_2$ at a 5 % significance level, the null hypothesis. (True/False).

9. The following figure reveals that there was no *Group* x *Method* interaction (please assume that every observed difference in the figures was statistically significant at 5 % significance level). (True/False).

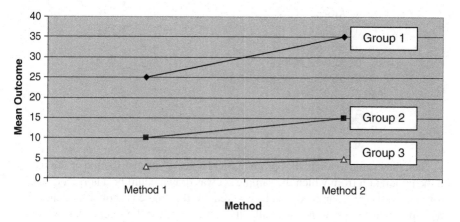

Mean responses of the outcomes for two different methods among the three study subgroups

10. An estimated multiple linear regression equation predicts the means of the dependent variable at particular values of the model's independent variables. (True or/False).
11. OR (odds ratio) is defined as the ratio of the two event probabilities of which the numerator is one group's event probability and the denominator is another group's (i.e., comparison group's) event probability. (True or/False).
12. In a 2×2 contingency table analysis setting, the alternative hypothesis of the Chi-square test can be directional. (True or/False).
13. Please explain "a statistic".
14. Please explain "a sampling distribution".
15. Please explain "a standard error".

9.2.2   Part B (15 Points): Questions 16.1–16.3

While interested in studying the performance on a mathematics proficiency test of a very large cohort of college freshmen in a developing country, a team of investigators had no knowledge about the population distribution of the performance scores. So, they gathered a pilot random sample of 100 individual scores and created the following stem-and-leaf plot and computed the mean and standard deviation (observed sample mean = 57 and the observed sample standard deviation = 17).

```
9  57
9  0
8  55666789
8  0012234
7  889
7  004
```

```
6  556689
6  0011344
5  566666778
5  012223334444
4  555555566668889999
4  0012222244
3  566789999
3  2234
2  6
```

Then they came to a statistics professor and asked if the distribution of the scores in the population from which the sample set was drawn could be a normal distribution. The professor examined it and answered "well … there is enough evidence that the population scores are not normally distributed because the sample data are clustered at two locations, i.e., bi-modal (having two modes)".

16.1. The sample median can be obtained from the information given to you: (True/ False). If you answered "True", please find out the median score. Otherwise please explain why you cannot obtain the sample median (5 points).
16.2. If a very large new random sample set is drawn (e.g., $n = 3,000$), the distribution of that new sample will approach to a normal (Gaussian) distribution: (True—Please explain why/False—Please explain why). (5 points).
16.3. If a very large number, m, of random sample sets with each individual sample size of 1,000 are independently drawn, then the distribution of those m independent sample means will probably form a symmetrical bell shape distribution: (True Please explain why/False—Please explain why) (5 points).

9.2.3   Part C (15 Points): Questions 17–19

The following descriptive statistics summarize the result of a small study of an effectiveness of a new intervention to improve elbow ROM (Range of Motion in degrees) among elderly men and women with previous elbow fracture.

	Control	Intervention A	Combined samples
Men	$N = 10$	$N = 10$	$N = 20$
	Mean = 30.10	Mean = 30.00	Mean = 30.05
	SD = 1.91	SD = 2.11	SD = 2.01
Women	$N = 30$	$N = 30$	$N = 60$
	Mean = 30.90	Mean = 36.40	Mean = 33.65
	SD = 1.91	SD = 2.27	SD = 2.10
Combined samples	$N = 40$	$N = 40$	$N = 80$
	Mean = 30.70	Mean = 34.80	Mean = 32.75
	SD = 1.91	SD = 2.23	SD = 2.08

17. Write an estimated regression equation that you would have obtained if a regression modeling (under the equal variance assumption) had been applied to women. Please let M_ROM (mean ROM) denote the dependent variable and let I_A denote the independent variable (a dummy variable indicating intervention A if its value = 1 and Control if 0), i.e., M_ROM = ( ) + ( )· I_A (5 points).
18. The intervention was not efficacious within men (statistical analysis test was performed, and the result was not significant). Please perform a directional t-test ($df = 58$) to examine whether or not the intervention was efficacious within women (please use a 5 % significance level and assume that the population variances are equal between the two groups) and make a statement that can appear in a clinical journal (5 points).
19. Was there an interaction? If so, please describe it; otherwise explain why the above information did not show an interaction (5 points).

9.2.4   Part D (10 Points): Questions 20–21

In a certain population, for a subject i ($i = 1, 2, 3, \ldots$, etc.), the measurement of Y is determined by the following linear model $Y_i = \beta_0 + \beta_1 X_i + \varepsilon_i$, where ε_i is a random error with mean 0. Y and X are both continuous variables and Y follows a normal distribution. The following equation is an estimated regression equation (using a sample data $n = 122$). The number in parentheses underneath the estimated regression slope coefficient is its standard error.

$$\hat{Y} = 100 + 2.25 \cdot X$$
$$(0.90)$$

Note: it was confirmed that the intercept β_0 was significantly greater than 0 ($p < 0.00001$), and the current estimate of 100 is clinically very meaningful.

20. Perform a z-test of which H_0: $\beta_1 = 0$ versus H_1: $\beta_1 > 0$, and write up a sentence that can go into a clinical journal results section. Please use a 5 % significance level (5 points).
21. Please construct a z-based 90 % CI around the β_1, and write up a sentence that can go into a clinical journal results section (5 points).

9.2.5   Part E (5 Points): Question 22

A small study showed that an estimated Pearson's product moment correlation coefficient between two continuous outcome variables using 12 pairs was 0.365, which was not significantly different from 0 at a 5 % significance level by the directional t-test (H_0: Population correlation coefficient $\rho = 0$ versus H_1: Population correlation coefficient $\rho > 0$).

There was another similar study result involving 22 pairs that showed $r=0.375$ without presenting a statistical test result.

22. Please perform a t-test of which the null and alternative hypotheses are H_0: Population correlation coefficient $\rho=0$ versus H_1: Population correlation coefficient $\rho>0$. Please use a 5 % significance level (df for the related statistical test $=20$). Please describe how you determined the significance of the result, and write up a sentence that can go into a clinical journal results section. Please do not include the explanation how you made your conclusion (i.e., do not make your answer like "... since p was less than ##, I rejected the null ...") (5 points).

9.2.6 Part F (20 Points): Questions 23–26

Please choose a *proper nonparametric method* for each analysis from the listed methods below.

23. Comparison of BMI (body mass index, i.e., [weight in pounds $\times 703$]/[height in inches^2]) distributions among three groups (5 points).
24. Test for examining whether or not there was a change in body weight between baseline and post 6 months life style modification intervention program offered to a group of obese subjects (5 points).
25. Test for an association between sex (male versus female) and smoking status (non-smokers versus smokers) (5 points).
26. Test for an association between age and heart rate (5 points).

   (a) Wilcoxon's signed-rank test
   (b) Mann–Whitney U-test (or Wilcoxon's rank sum test)
   (c) Kruskal–Wallis test
   (d) Friedman's test
   (e) Chi-square test for independence
   (f) McNemar's test for matched pairs
   (g) Spearman's rank correlation

Chapter 10
Probability Distribution of Standard Normal Distribution

H. Lee, *Foundations of Applied Statistical Methods*, DOI 10.1007/978-3-319-02402-8_10,   145
© Springer International Publishing Switzerland 2014

Table 10.1 Cumulative probability distribution of standard normal distribution

Cumulative probability	Evaluated from negative infinity to	Cumulative probability	Evaluated from negative infinity to	Cumulative probability	Evaluated from negative infinity to	Cumulative probability	Evaluated from negative infinity to	Cumulative probability	Evaluated from negative infinity to
0.005	−2.5758	0.200	−0.8416	0.400	−0.2533	0.600	0.2533	0.800	0.8416
0.010	−2.3263	0.205	−0.8239	0.405	−0.2404	0.605	0.2663	0.805	0.8596
0.015	−2.1701	0.210	−0.8064	0.410	−0.2275	0.610	0.2793	0.810	0.8779
0.020	−2.0537	0.215	−0.7892	0.415	−0.2147	0.615	0.2924	0.815	0.8965
0.025	−1.9600	0.220	−0.7722	0.420	−0.2019	0.620	0.3055	0.820	0.9154
0.030	−1.8808	0.225	−0.7554	0.425	−0.1891	0.625	0.3186	0.825	0.9346
0.035	−1.8119	0.230	−0.7388	0.430	−0.1764	0.630	0.3319	0.830	0.9542
0.040	−1.7507	0.235	−0.7225	0.435	−0.1637	0.635	0.3451	0.835	0.9741
0.045	−1.6954	0.240	−0.7063	0.440	−0.1510	0.640	0.3585	0.840	0.9945
0.050	−1.6449	0.245	−0.6903	0.445	−0.1383	0.645	0.3719	0.845	1.0152
0.055	−1.5982	0.250	−0.6745	0.450	−0.1257	0.650	0.3853	0.850	1.0364
0.060	−1.5548	0.255	−0.6588	0.455	−0.1130	0.655	0.3989	0.855	1.0581
0.065	−1.5141	0.260	−0.6433	0.460	−0.1004	0.660	0.4125	0.860	1.0803
0.070	−1.4758	0.265	−0.6280	0.465	−0.0878	0.665	0.4261	0.865	1.1031
0.075	−1.4395	0.270	−0.6128	0.470	−0.0753	0.670	0.4399	0.870	1.1264
0.080	−1.4051	0.275	−0.5978	0.475	−0.0627	0.675	0.4538	0.875	1.1503
0.085	−1.3722	0.280	−0.5828	0.480	−0.0502	0.680	0.4677	0.880	1.1750
0.090	−1.3408	0.285	−0.5681	0.485	−0.0376	0.685	0.4817	0.885	1.2004
0.095	−1.3106	0.290	−0.5534	0.490	−0.0251	0.690	0.4959	0.890	1.2265
0.100	−1.2816	0.295	−0.5388	0.495	−0.0125	0.695	0.5101	0.895	1.2536
0.105	−1.2536	0.300	−0.5244	0.500	0.0000	0.700	0.5244	0.900	1.2816
0.110	−1.2265	0.305	−0.5101	0.505	0.0125	0.705	0.5388	0.905	1.3106
		0.310	−0.4959	0.510	0.0251	0.710	0.5534	0.910	1.3408

p	z	p	z	p	z	p	z	p	z
0.115	−1.2004	0.315	−0.4817	0.515	0.0376	0.715	0.5681	0.915	1.3722
0.120	−1.1750	0.320	−0.4677	0.520	0.0502	0.720	0.5828	0.920	1.4051
0.125	−1.1503	0.325	−0.4538	0.525	0.0627	0.725	0.5978	0.925	1.4395
0.130	−1.1264	0.330	−0.4399	0.530	0.0753	0.730	0.6128	0.930	1.4758
0.135	−1.1031	0.335	−0.4261	0.535	0.0878	0.735	0.6280	0.935	1.5141
0.140	−1.0803	0.340	−0.4125	0.540	0.1004	0.740	0.6433	0.940	1.5548
0.145	−1.0581	0.345	−0.3989	0.545	0.1130	0.745	0.6588	0.945	1.5982
0.150	−1.0364	0.350	−0.3853	0.550	0.1257	0.750	0.6745	0.950	1.6449
0.155	−1.0152	0.355	−0.3719	0.555	0.1383	0.755	0.6903	0.955	1.6954
0.160	−0.9945	0.360	−0.3585	0.560	0.1510	0.760	0.7063	0.960	1.7507
0.165	−0.9741	0.365	−0.3451	0.565	0.1637	0.765	0.7225	0.965	1.8119
0.170	−0.9542	0.370	−0.3319	0.570	0.1764	0.770	0.7388	0.970	1.8808
0.175	−0.9346	0.375	−0.3186	0.575	0.1891	0.775	0.7554	0.975	1.9600
0.180	−0.9154	0.380	−0.3055	0.580	0.2019	0.780	0.7722	0.980	2.0537
0.185	−0.8965	0.385	−0.2924	0.585	0.2147	0.785	0.7892	0.985	2.1701
0.190	−0.8779	0.390	−0.2793	0.590	0.2275	0.790	0.8064	0.990	2.3263
0.195	−0.8596	0.395	−0.2663	0.595	0.2404	0.795	0.8239	0.995	2.5758

Chapter 11
Percentiles of *t*-Distributions

Table 11.1 Absolute value of t statistic (i.e., |t|) given *df* and tail (both upper and lower tails) probability

df	p=0.0005	p=0.001	p=0.025	p=0.05	p=0.075	p=0.1
2	44.7046	31.5991	6.2053	4.3027	3.4428	2.9200
3	16.3263	12.9240	4.1765	3.1824	2.6808	2.3534
4	10.3063	8.6103	3.4954	2.7764	2.3921	2.1318
5	7.9757	6.8688	3.1634	2.5706	2.2423	2.0150
6	6.7883	5.9588	2.9687	2.4469	2.1510	1.9432
7	6.0818	5.4079	2.8412	2.3646	2.0897	1.8946
8	5.6174	5.0413	2.7515	2.3060	2.0458	1.8595
9	5.2907	4.7809	2.6850	2.2622	2.0127	1.8331
10	5.0490	4.5869	2.6338	2.2281	1.9870	1.8125
11	4.8633	4.4370	2.5931	2.2010	1.9663	1.7959
12	4.7165	4.3178	2.5600	2.1788	1.9494	1.7823
13	4.5975	4.2208	2.5326	2.1604	1.9354	1.7709
14	4.4992	4.1405	2.5096	2.1448	1.9235	1.7613
15	4.4166	4.0728	2.4899	2.1314	1.9132	1.7531
16	4.3463	4.0150	2.4729	2.1199	1.9044	1.7459
17	4.2858	3.9651	2.4581	2.1098	1.8966	1.7396
18	4.2332	3.9216	2.4450	2.1009	1.8898	1.7341
19	4.1869	3.8834	2.4334	2.0930	1.8837	1.7291
20	4.1460	3.8495	2.4231	2.0860	1.8783	1.7247
21	4.1096	3.8193	2.4138	2.0796	1.8734	1.7207
22	4.0769	3.7921	2.4055	2.0739	1.8690	1.7171
23	4.0474	3.7676	2.3979	2.0687	1.8649	1.7139
24	4.0207	3.7454	2.3909	2.0639	1.8613	1.7109
25	3.9964	3.7251	2.3846	2.0595	1.8579	1.7081
26	3.9742	3.7066	2.3788	2.0555	1.8548	1.7056
27	3.9538	3.6896	2.3734	2.0518	1.8519	1.7033
28	3.9351	3.6739	2.3685	2.0484	1.8493	1.7011
29	3.9177	3.6594	2.3638	2.0452	1.8468	1.6991

(continued)

H. Lee, *Foundations of Applied Statistical Methods*, DOI 10.1007/978-3-319-02402-8_11,   149
© Springer International Publishing Switzerland 2014

Table 11.1 (continued)

df	$p=0.0005$	$p=0.001$	$p=0.025$	$p=0.05$	$p=0.075$	$p=0.1$
30	3.9016	3.6460	2.3596	2.0423	1.8445	1.6973
31	3.8867	3.6335	2.3556	2.0395	1.8424	1.6955
32	3.8728	3.6218	2.3518	2.0369	1.8404	1.6939
33	3.8598	3.6109	2.3483	2.0345	1.8385	1.6924
34	3.8476	3.6007	2.3451	2.0322	1.8368	1.6909
35	3.8362	3.5911	2.3420	2.0301	1.8351	1.6896
50	3.7231	3.4960	2.3109	2.0086	1.8184	1.6759
75	3.6391	3.4250	2.2873	1.9921	1.8056	1.6654
100	3.5983	3.3905	2.2757	1.9840	1.7992	1.6602

Chapter 12
Upper 95th and 99th Percentiles of Chi-Square Distributions

H. Lee, *Foundations of Applied Statistical Methods*, DOI 10.1007/978-3-319-02402-8_12,   151
© Springer International Publishing Switzerland 2014

Table 12.1 Upper 95th (5 % upper tail) and 99th (1 % upper tail) percentiles of chi-square distributions

df	95th (5 % upper tail)	99th (1 % upper tail)
1	3.84	6.63
2	5.99	9.21
3	7.81	11.34
4	9.49	13.28
5	11.07	15.09
6	12.59	16.81
7	14.07	18.48
8	15.51	20.09
9	16.92	21.67
10	18.31	23.21
11	19.68	24.72
12	21.03	26.22
13	22.36	27.69
14	23.68	29.14
15	25.00	30.58
16	26.30	32.00
17	27.59	33.41
18	28.87	34.81
19	30.14	36.19
20	31.41	37.57
21	32.67	38.93
22	33.92	40.29
23	35.17	41.64
24	36.42	42.98
25	37.65	44.31
26	38.89	45.64
27	40.11	46.96
28	41.34	48.28
29	42.56	49.59
30	43.77	50.89
35	49.80	57.34
40	55.76	63.69
45	61.66	69.96
50	67.50	76.15
75	96.22	106.39
100	124.34	135.81

Chapter 13
Upper 95th Percentiles of *F*-Distributions

Table 13.1 Upper 95th percentiles of *F*-distributions

df_2	df_1									
	1	2	3	4	5	6	7	8	9	10
2	18.51	19.00	19.16	19.25	19.30	19.33	19.35	19.37	19.38	19.40
3	10.13	9.55	9.28	9.12	9.01	8.94	8.89	8.85	8.81	8.79
4	7.71	6.94	6.59	6.39	6.26	6.16	6.09	6.04	6.00	5.96
5	6.61	5.79	5.41	5.19	5.05	4.95	4.88	4.82	4.77	4.74
6	5.99	5.14	4.76	4.53	4.39	4.28	4.21	4.15	4.10	4.06
7	5.59	4.74	4.35	4.12	3.97	3.87	3.79	3.73	3.68	3.64
8	5.32	4.46	4.07	3.84	3.69	3.58	3.50	3.44	3.39	3.35
9	5.12	4.26	3.86	3.63	3.48	3.37	3.29	3.23	3.18	3.14
10	4.96	4.10	3.71	3.48	3.33	3.22	3.14	3.07	3.02	2.98
11	4.84	3.98	3.59	3.36	3.20	3.09	3.01	2.95	2.90	2.85
12	4.75	3.89	3.49	3.26	3.11	3.00	2.91	2.85	2.80	2.75
13	4.67	3.81	3.41	3.18	3.03	2.92	2.83	2.77	2.71	2.67
14	4.60	3.74	3.34	3.11	2.96	2.85	2.76	2.70	2.65	2.60
15	4.54	3.68	3.29	3.06	2.90	2.79	2.71	2.64	2.59	2.54
16	4.49	3.63	3.24	3.01	2.85	2.74	2.66	2.59	2.54	2.49
17	4.45	3.59	3.20	2.96	2.81	2.70	2.61	2.55	2.49	2.45
18	4.41	3.55	3.16	2.93	2.77	2.66	2.58	2.51	2.46	2.41
19	4.38	3.52	3.13	2.90	2.74	2.63	2.54	2.48	2.42	2.38
20	4.35	3.49	3.10	2.87	2.71	2.60	2.51	2.45	2.39	2.35
21	4.32	3.47	3.07	2.84	2.68	2.57	2.49	2.42	2.37	2.32
22	4.30	3.44	3.05	2.82	2.66	2.55	2.46	2.40	2.34	2.30
23	4.28	3.42	3.03	2.80	2.64	2.53	2.44	2.37	2.32	2.27
24	4.26	3.40	3.01	2.78	2.62	2.51	2.42	2.36	2.30	2.25
25	4.24	3.39	2.99	2.76	2.60	2.49	2.40	2.34	2.28	2.24
26	4.23	3.37	2.98	2.74	2.59	2.47	2.39	2.32	2.27	2.22
27	4.21	3.35	2.96	2.73	2.57	2.46	2.37	2.31	2.25	2.20
28	4.20	3.34	2.95	2.71	2.56	2.45	2.36	2.29	2.24	2.19
29	4.18	3.33	2.93	2.70	2.55	2.43	2.35	2.28	2.22	2.18
30	4.17	3.32	2.92	2.69	2.53	2.42	2.33	2.27	2.21	2.16

(continued)

H. Lee, *Foundations of Applied Statistical Methods*, DOI 10.1007/978-3-319-02402-8_13, 153
© Springer International Publishing Switzerland 2014

Table 13.1   (continued)

df_2	df_1									
	1	2	3	4	5	6	7	8	9	10
35	4.12	3.27	2.87	2.64	2.49	2.37	2.29	2.22	2.16	2.11
40	4.08	3.23	2.84	2.61	2.45	2.34	2.25	2.18	2.12	2.08
45	4.06	3.20	2.81	2.58	2.42	2.31	2.22	2.15	2.10	2.05
50	4.03	3.18	2.79	2.56	2.40	2.29	2.20	2.13	2.07	2.03
55	4.02	3.16	2.77	2.54	2.38	2.27	2.18	2.11	2.06	2.01
60	4.00	3.15	2.76	2.53	2.37	2.25	2.17	2.10	2.04	1.99
75	3.97	3.12	2.73	2.49	2.34	2.22	2.13	2.06	2.01	1.96
100	3.94	3.09	2.70	2.46	2.31	2.19	2.10	2.03	1.97	1.93

df_1—numerator df
df_2—denominator df

Chapter 14
Upper 99th Percentiles of F-Distributions

Table 14.1 Upper 99th percentiles of F-distributions

df_2	df_1									
	1	2	3	4	5	6	7	8	9	10
2	98.50	99.00	99.17	99.25	99.30	99.33	99.36	99.37	99.39	99.40
3	34.12	30.82	29.46	28.71	28.24	27.91	27.67	27.49	27.35	27.23
4	21.20	18.00	16.69	15.98	15.52	15.21	14.98	14.80	14.66	14.55
5	16.26	13.27	12.06	11.39	10.97	10.67	10.46	10.29	10.16	10.05
6	13.75	10.92	9.78	9.15	8.75	8.47	8.26	8.10	7.98	7.87
7	12.25	9.55	8.45	7.85	7.46	7.19	6.99	6.84	6.72	6.62
8	11.26	8.65	7.59	7.01	6.63	6.37	6.18	6.03	5.91	5.81
9	10.56	8.02	6.99	6.42	6.06	5.80	5.61	5.47	5.35	5.26
10	10.04	7.56	6.55	5.99	5.64	5.39	5.20	5.06	4.94	4.85
11	9.65	7.21	6.22	5.67	5.32	5.07	4.89	4.74	4.63	4.54
12	9.33	6.93	5.95	5.41	5.06	4.82	4.64	4.50	4.39	4.30
13	9.07	6.70	5.74	5.21	4.86	4.62	4.44	4.30	4.19	4.10
14	8.86	6.51	5.56	5.04	4.69	4.46	4.28	4.14	4.03	3.94
15	8.68	6.36	5.42	4.89	4.56	4.32	4.14	4.00	3.89	3.80
16	8.53	6.23	5.29	4.77	4.44	4.20	4.03	3.89	3.78	3.69
17	8.40	6.11	5.18	4.67	4.34	4.10	3.93	3.79	3.68	3.59
18	8.29	6.01	5.09	4.58	4.25	4.01	3.84	3.71	3.60	3.51
19	8.18	5.93	5.01	4.50	4.17	3.94	3.77	3.63	3.52	3.43
20	8.10	5.85	4.94	4.43	4.10	3.87	3.70	3.56	3.46	3.37
21	8.02	5.78	4.87	4.37	4.04	3.81	3.64	3.51	3.40	3.31
22	7.95	5.72	4.82	4.31	3.99	3.76	3.59	3.45	3.35	3.26
23	7.88	5.66	4.76	4.26	3.94	3.71	3.54	3.41	3.30	3.21
24	7.82	5.61	4.72	4.22	3.90	3.67	3.50	3.36	3.26	3.17
25	7.77	5.57	4.68	4.18	3.85	3.63	3.46	3.32	3.22	3.13
26	7.72	5.53	4.64	4.14	3.82	3.59	3.42	3.29	3.18	3.09
27	7.68	5.49	4.60	4.11	3.78	3.56	3.39	3.26	3.15	3.06
28	7.64	5.45	4.57	4.07	3.75	3.53	3.36	3.23	3.12	3.03
29	7.60	5.42	4.54	4.04	3.73	3.50	3.33	3.20	3.09	3.00

(continued)

H. Lee, *Foundations of Applied Statistical Methods*, DOI 10.1007/978-3-319-02402-8_14, 155
© Springer International Publishing Switzerland 2014

Table 14.1 (continued)

df_2	df_1									
	1	2	3	4	5	6	7	8	9	10
30	7.56	5.39	4.51	4.02	3.70	3.47	3.30	3.17	3.07	2.98
35	7.42	5.27	4.40	3.91	3.59	3.37	3.20	3.07	2.96	2.88
40	7.31	5.18	4.31	3.83	3.51	3.29	3.12	2.99	2.89	2.80
45	7.23	5.11	4.25	3.77	3.45	3.23	3.07	2.94	2.83	2.74
50	7.17	5.06	4.20	3.72	3.41	3.19	3.02	2.89	2.78	2.70
55	7.12	5.01	4.16	3.68	3.37	3.15	2.98	2.85	2.75	2.66
60	7.08	4.98	4.13	3.65	3.34	3.12	2.95	2.82	2.72	2.63
75	6.99	4.90	4.05	3.58	3.27	3.05	2.89	2.76	2.65	2.57
100	6.90	4.82	3.98	3.51	3.21	2.99	2.82	2.69	2.59	2.50

df_1—numerator df
df_2—denominator df

Chapter 15
Sample Sizes for Independent Samples *t*-Tests

Table 15.1 Sample size per group for two-group independent samples *t*-test (normal approximation)

Effect size = (mean difference/ common SD)	Alpha = 0.01 (two-sided)		Alpha = 0.05 (two-sided)	
	Power = 0.8	Power = 0.9	Power = 0.8	Power = 0.9
0.25	373	476	251	336
0.30	259	330	174	233
0.35	190	242	128	171
0.40	145	185	98	131
0.45	115	146	77	103
0.50	93	119	62	84
0.55	77	98	51	69
0.60	64	82	43	58
0.65	55	70	37	49
0.70	47	60	32	42
0.75	41	52	27	37
0.80	36	46	24	32
0.85	32	41	21	29
0.90	28	36	19	25
0.95	25	32	17	23
1.00	23	29	15	21
1.05	21	26	14	19
1.10	19	24	12	17
1.15	17	22	11	15
1.20	16	20	10	14
1.25	14	19	10	13

H. Lee, *Foundations of Applied Statistical Methods*, DOI 10.1007/978-3-319-02402-8_15,   157
© Springer International Publishing Switzerland 2014

ERRATUM

Foundations of Applied Statistical Methods

Hang Lee

H. Lee, *Foundations of Applied Statistical Methods*, DOI 10.1007/978-3-319-02402-8,
© Springer International Publishing Switzerland 2014

DOI 10.1007/978-3-319-02402-8_16

The author's correct affiliation is Massachusetts General Hospital Biostatistics Center and Harvard Medical School, Boston, Massachusetts.

Index

A
Accuracy, 48–50
Alpha (α), 41, 49
Alternative hypothesis, 39
Analysis of variance (ANOVA), 75–77
Association, 18, 19

B
Bayesian inference, 54–56
Bayes' rule, 54, 56
Beta (β), 49
Between group sum of square, 76
Bias, 50
Binary (dichotomous) outcome, 25, 28, 95, 96,
        105, 106, 110
Binomial distribution, 21, 25–28,
Bonferroni's correction, 81
Box-and-Whiskers plot, 17–18

C
Categorical data, 1, 3, 105
Censored survival times, 121–124
Censoring, 121
Central Limit Theorem, 35–37
Central tendency, 35
Chi-square test, 106–109
Coefficient of variation (CV), 14, 15
Confidence interval, 50–54
Contingency table, 19–20, 105–112
Continuity correction, 108
Continuous outcome, 2
Correlation coefficient, 18, 19, 87–88

Count outcome, 2
Cox–Mantel test, 124

D
Degrees of freedom (df), 37, 38
Density, 21–22
Dependent variable, 75, 89
Descriptive statistics, 8–17
Deviation, 9–11
Directional test, 41
Distribution-free methods, 114

E
Effect size, 127–129
Error sum of square, 75, 76
Error term, 89
Estimation, 35
Expected frequency, 107, 108

F
F-distribution, 78–81
Fisher's exact test, 109–110
F-test, 77–81

G
Gaussian distribution (normal distribution),
        21–25, 27
Generalized linear model,
        98–99
General linear model, 98–99

Printed in the United States
By Bookmasters